GARLAND STUDIES IN

AMERICAN POPULAR HISTORY AND CULTURE

edited by

JEROME NADELHAFT
UNIVERSITY OF MAINE

A GARLAND SERIES

Garland Studies in American Popular History and Culture

Jerome Nadelhaft, series editor

Seduction, Prostitution, and Moral Reform in New York, 1830–1860
Larry Whiteaker

Hollywood's Vision of Team Sports: Heroes, Race, and Gender
Deborah V. Tudor

The Flamingo in the Garden: American Yard Art and the Vernacular Landscape
Colleen J. Sheehy

Textual Vehicles: The Automobile in American Literature
Roger N. Casey

Film and the Nuclear Age: Representing Cultural Anxiety
Toni A. Perrine

Lesbian and Gay Memphis: Building Communities Behind the Magnolia Curtain
Daneel Buring

Making Villains, Making Heroes: Joseph R. McCarthy, Martin Luther King, Jr., and the Politics of American Memory
Gary Daynes

America Under Construction: Boundaries and Identities in Popular Culture
Kristi S. Long and Matthew Nadelhaft, editors

AIDS, Social Change, and Theater: Performance as Protest
Cindy J. Kistenberg

"When the Spirit Says Sing!": The Role of Freedom Songs in the Civil Rights Movement
Kerran L. Sanger

African American Nationalist Literature of the 1960s: Pens of Fire
Sandra Hollin Flowers

The Rehabilitation of Richard Nixon: The Media's Effect on Collective Memory
Thomas J. Johnson

Chicano Images: Refiguring Ethnicity in Mainstream Film
Christine List

At a Theater or Drive-in Near You: The History, Culture, and Politics of the American Exploitation Film
Randall Clark

Lolita in Peyton Place: Highbrow, Lowbrow, and Middlebrow Novels of the 1950s
Ruth Wood

Contra Dance Choreography: A Reflection of Social Change
Mary Dart

Public Discourse and Academic Inquiry
William Craig Rice

The Intellectual Origins of Mass Parties and Mass Schools in the Jacksonian Era: Creating a Conformed Citizenry
Julie M. Walsh

Early American Women Dramatists, 1775–1860
Zoe Detsi-Diamanti

Understanding Elvis: Southern Roots vs. Star Image
Susan M. Doll

Gynecology and Textuality: Popular Representations of Reproductive Technology
Chloé Diepenbrock

GYNECOLOGY AND TEXTUALITY

Popular Representations of Reproductive Technology

CHLOÉ DIEPENBROCK

GARLAND PUBLISHING, INC.
A MEMBER OF THE TAYLOR & FRANCIS GROUP
NEW YORK & LONDON / 1998

Library of Congress Cataloging-in-Publication Data

Diepenbrock, Chloé, 1955–
Gynecology and textuality : popular representations of reproductive technology / Chloé Diepenbrock.
p. cm. — (Garland studies in American popular history and culture)
Includes bibliographical references and index.
ISBN 0-8153-3222-X (alk. paper)
1. Human reproductive technology—United States—History. 2. Gynecology—United States—History. 3. Medicine—United States—History—19th century. 4. Medicine—United States—History—20th century. 5. Medicine in literature. 6. Popular culture. I. Title. II. Series.
[DNLM: 1. Reproductive Techniques—history—United States. 2. Gynecology—history—United States. 3. History of Medicine, 19th cent.—United States. 4. History of Medicine, 20th cent.—United States. 5. Medicine in Literature. 6. Periodicals. WQ 11 AA1 D562g 1998]
RG133.5.D54 1998
618.1'00973—dc21
DNLM/DLC
for Library of Congress

98-41890

Printed on acid-free, 250-year-life paper
Manufactured in the United States of America

This book is dedicated to my mother, Marjorie Gossage Schoorl Diepenbrock and my son, Donald Jerome. Thank you both for the inspiration and the patience.

Contents

Figures

Acknowledgments

Many people made it possible for me to write this book. I want to thank Donald Newman for helping me to formulate the idea of the gynecological case history and then helping me to find 19th-century texts. Jody Bosworth, Dagmar Corrigan, Simone Gers, Kathy Landis, and Mac McGinty lent their scholarly support, editing work, and sometimes even baby-sitting so I could write. Without the five of you, this book would not exist.

On a different note, I would like to acknowledge the inspiration provided to me by my mother. The mother of twelve surviving children, she made birth look easy. Her remarkable mothering is what sparked my interest in the subject of birth. Her strength, determination, and spirit have shown me that when you really want something you can achieve it if you work hard enough.

Chloé Diepenbrock

Gynecology and Textuality

CHAPTER ONE

Gynecology in Context

> Man is
> the symbol-using (symbol-making, symbol-misusing) animal
> inventor of the negative (or moralized by the negative)
> separated from his natural condition by instruments of his own
> making
> goaded by the spirit of hierarchy (or moved by the sense of order)
> and rotten with perfection. (Burke *Language* 16)

Kenneth Burke's "Definition of Man" is based on the distinctly human ability to use a symbolic code to compose and transmit meaning.[1] This ability has also facilitated the development of technology, a relationship Burke draws in the third clause of the definition: the symbolic instrument of language, together with the physical implements it allows us to conceptualize, distances human motivation from the basic needs of food, shelter, and sex. The refined technologies of the twentieth century depend upon the use of the symbolic code not only for their existence, but also for their dissemination.

Of the many areas in which one could explore this relationship between the ability to symbolize and our twentieth-century technologies, I wish to look at a sub-genre that has become extremely popular and influential in the latter half of the century: the gynecological case history. This dramatic narrative presents birth stories in the popular media to a variety of audiences. Those who read women's service magazines, commentary journals, news magazines, newspapers, and fiction are treated to different versions of the gynecological case history. In the women's magazine, where birth stories have the widest audience, the case history is easily adapted to serve as a highly persuasive tool for the practices it announces and promotes. [2] Because audience sympathy and identification are so easily evoked in this venue, the gynecological case history plays an important role in advancing the technologies that have been created to assist reproduction and genetic manipulation.

The response to these mini-dramas is always strong, whether positive or negative. Women aspiring to motherhood may find themselves identifying with the women whose stories fill the pages of the *Good Housekeeping* magazine they pick up at the check-out stand. Readers interested in social critique will find arguments for and against every aspect of reproductive technologies in the *Commentary* or *National Review* they place on their coffee tables or the newspapers and magazines they read at the breakfast table.

This mixed reception is very understandable. Parenthood is both a biological and social imperative. Aside from our obvious need to propagate our species, our social nature drives us to create and maintain cooperative family units for the emotional support we need to survive. We gain many benefits from parenthood. Our children allow us to relive childhood, a process that provides us with the opportunity to learn about ourselves and to mature emotionally, intellectually and spiritually. Children's unconditional love and dependence give our lives purpose and meaning. Reproduction also represents a rite of passage for both men and women. Fertility makes us feel whole and capable. Men who father children have proven their manhood biologically. Women who conceive, gestate, and deliver children demonstrate the strength and endurance unique to our gender. The healthy, happy, and productive children we all aspire to raise are our greatest contribution to our society. Some parents' dreams for their children go beyond successful socialization; they hope to parent a child who will win the Noble Prize, become President, score the winning touchdown in the Superbowl, travel to Mars, or discover the cure for AIDS. Finally, in our old age, we hope that our children will give us comfort, support, and care.

Though some are perfectly happy raising adopted children, for others, the drive to reproduce is only satisfied by a genetically-related child. We want to reproduce our husband's winning smile or our wife's enchanting laugh. Having a genetically-related child also ensures the continuation of our hereditary line in the gene pool. To satisfy, and one could argue, to reinforce this need for a genetic connection, reproductive technologies have been developed by our scientifically oriented society. Such services have in fact brought joy to many aspiring parents. Between 1985 and 1993, live births from in vitro fertilization rose from 1,200 to 8,700 (Neumann "Should health" 1215).

Unfortunately, assisted reproduction brings with it a host of accompanying ethical problems that must be considered if we wish to be fully informed about how the scientific production of children will change the shape of our society. One of the most important social changes wrought by reproductive technologies is the fragmentation of parenthood. Previously, one could become a genetic or an adoptive parent. With egg donation and surrogacy, both "traditional" and "gestational,"[3] we have divided motherhood into three separate functions: genetic, gestational, and social. With sperm donation, we have divided fatherhood into two separate functions: genetic and social. This fragmentation introduces a hierarchy of parenthood that confuses legal decisions, complicates social relationships, and creates untenable moral dilemmas.

Several well-publicized cases have illustrated some of the legal and social issues that fertility procedures create. When Marybeth Whitehead-Gould sued for custody of Baby M, she was fighting to break a surrogacy contract that gave all rights to her genetic and biological daughter to the child's genetic father, William Stern, and his wife, Elizabeth. Following traditional legal practice, the court determined that the child would be better off with the more affluent Sterns and awarded them custody. This decision was overturned on appeal and Whitehead-Gould now has visitation rights with her daughter. The second decision took into account the fact that Baby M was Whitehead-Gould's genetic and gestational daughter and that, despite the contract, she found it impossible to relinquish the bond she had with the baby. Once the New Jersey courts recognized the problematic nature of surrogacy contracts, legislation was passed to ban the practice of contracting motherhood.

In California, where there are no regulations for the surrogacy industry, Anna Johnson, serving as a "gestational surrogate" for Michael and Crispina Calvert, claimed she too had bonded with the child she carried and sued for custody. The judge ruled her a "genetic stranger" and awarded custody to the Calverts because they had supplied the genetic material. Based on this case, genetics would appear to be an important deciding factor in custody disputes, but the genetic relationship is not always a clear determinant of who will be awarded rights to a child. Egg and sperm donation complicate legal decisions. When people donate genetic material so that others can use it to reproduce, can they then make later claims to the offspring? In this type of case, intentions tend to prevail in legal decisions. Determining what is best for a child becomes complicated, however, when genetically unrelated parents nurture a child who is later discovered to "belong" genetically to someone else. This is the case with many couples who were treated at the UC-Riverside fertility clinic. Some of the doctors were accused of selling fertilized eggs to couples who were unsuccessful at producing their own. At least one suit has been filed to gain custody of four-year old twins whose genetic material may have belonged to one couple while they were gestated and nurtured by another. Intentions are difficult to sort out in a case such as this. A 1997 child support suit illustrates the extent to which we have divided parenthood. Jaycee Buzzanca was created using donors for both the egg and sperm and a contract mother for gestation. After her birth and before he adopted her, the intended social father, John Buzzanca, changed his mind. The social mother, his wife, sued for child support and a California court found him not responsible because he lacked a biological connection to the child. The social mother was termed the "'temporary custodial person'" by the court (Goodman 6C).

Another complicated scenario arises when a genetically unrelated partner—either homosexual or heterosexual—nurtures a child but loses custody after the relationship fails. In this situation, a social relationship that has been in place for the crucial first years of a child's life could be terminated, depriving the child of his/her primary caregiver. Grandparents could conceivably sue for visitation rights on the grounds that they never agreed to give up their rights to a child their daughter conceived as a surrogate. These scenarios indicate that intentions alone will not resolve such situations. Clearly, legal definitions have not caught up with the many permutations of parenthood made possible by reproductive technologies.

Another problematic result of assisted reproduction is financial burden. People spend their savings, mortgage their homes, and go deeply into debt to finance their quest for parenthood. The price tag on the least expensive IVF baby is $67,000 for one attempt and $114,000 for six attempts (Neumann, Gharib, and Weinstein 242). For older women and for men with infertility problems, the sticker price increases dramatically: $160,000 for just one attempt and as much as $800,000 for six attempts (241). Women make this investment with the belief that the procedures they will endure are effective. However, older women, who are arguably the most likely to be seeking help, spend more money, incur more physical risk, and are least likely to succeed. Recent medical research indicates that IVF treatment is most effective with the first attempt; with subsequent attempts, the rate of conception actually goes down (Templeton, Morris, and Parslow 1406). These same researchers also found that age is the most significant factor in the success or failure of in vitro technologies: "The success rates at ages 40 and 45 are only 7% and 2%" (1406). Multiple births also raise the financial costs of assisted reproduction (Brownlee 93).

Along with legal and financial problems, reproductive technologies exact a physical toll on those who participate in them. In addition to the expected side effects of the powerful hormones used by fertility services, medical researchers are looking into a possible connection between the use of these drugs and an increased risk of breast and ovarian cancers (Venn, Watson, Lumley, Giles, et al. 995). While the jury is still out on this connection, typical side effects include a host of other physical dangers ranging from infections and hyperstimulation of the ovaries, to high-risk pregnancies brought on by the increased chance of carrying multiple fetuses to term (Kershner 31). In addition to the risk to the mother, multiple-births—up 214% in the U.S. since 1980 (Cimones 12A)—pose enormous risks to the fetuses. The nation was pleasantly shocked last November when Bobby McCaughey gave birth to seven fetuses she gestated without any apparent birth defects or complications. Not every mother of multiples is so lucky, however. Medical statistics indicate that babies that are the product of multiple births are 10 times more likely to be born prematurely and with low birth weights (Kershner 31), two to three times more likely to suffer from spina bifida and heart abnormalities (Cohen 20), 47 times more likely to have cerebral palsy (Brownlee 93), and four times more likely to die (Kershner 31). In the United States, the incidence of multiple births is 1 in 250 with in vitro, and 1 in 13 with GIFT ("Fertility Clinics" 53).

Even when multiples are carried without injury, the challenge of parenting and providing for three, four, five, six, or seven same-age children is monumental. The McCaugheys have been blessed with round-the-clock shift help from their church congregation; without this assistance, they would be trying to feed and diaper seven babies without depriving them of the attention they need. Seven infants represent approximately 70 diaper changes a day, 40-50 bottles per day, and countless hours of bathing, dressing, rocking, and nurturing. Raising multiples is also a financial challenge that has become enough of an issue to warrant discussions in *Money* and *Finance* magazines. Births like the McCaughey septuplets are unusual enough to inspire contributions from corporate America: a new van, a "lifetime" supply of diapers, food, clothing, a free college education for each child, and a new home. Parents of triplets and quadruplets, who are becoming old news, can't expect to receive this kind of help.

Perhaps the most troubling dilemmas created by reproductive technologies are moral. Because of the great cost—physical and financial—of extracting eggs for in vitro fertilization, it has become common practice to induce ovulation of several eggs, then fertilize and freeze any "extras." Hundreds of thousands of embryos have been created across the world, remaining in a state of frozen animation in embryo banks. Custody battles have been waged, with one spouse seeking to implant the embryos and the other wishing to thaw them out and dispose of them. The legal status of frozen embryos is uncertain; are they human life or genetic property? Fertility personnel in Britain recently thawed out more than 3000 frozen embryos after a law was passed requiring clinics to dispose of unclaimed embryos more than five years old (White 4). Is this murder? Those who believe that life begins at conception would argue that it is, and that the creation and destruction of life in this manner is as irresponsible as abortion. On the other hand, if frozen embryos do not have full human rights, then they are fair game for medical research. Indeed, just four years ago, scientists were partially successful at cloning some defective embryos in their laboratory. Since Scottish scientists cloned a lamb in February, 1997, several bills banning cloning have been introduced in the legislature, but the United States Senate just defeated the most recent one after an effective lobbying effort by biomedical researchers (Gianelli 51).

The United States has no laws regulating how many embryos are implanted during an in vitro cycle. Because it has become increasingly common to implant up to four or five at a time, women are then faced with the choice of carrying all of the fetuses at great risk or undergoing selective reduction: aborting one or more so the others will survive. For a woman who has waited for years to become pregnant, and who without doubt wants her babies, such a choice must be agonizing.

A less obvious moral question is whether it is unethical to hire women to serve as surrogates when they may be motivated by financial gain. Disadvantaged women may view the fees paid for surrogacy and egg donation as an attractive path to greater financial security and, because of this, ignore the emotional and physical risks involved. Feminist commentators have speculated that we will eventually develop a breeder class of women, valued only for their ability to gestate. The practice of gestating a child only to give it to other parents also involves a great deal of psychological risk. Marybeth Whitehead-Gould found she could not honor her contract. Other women who have functioned as contract mothers have also denounced the practice, most notably a woman called "Elizabeth Kane"[4] who began by advertising the joys of surrogacy and later became one of its harshest critics.

The practice of surrogacy can be psychologically damaging for everyone involved, especially if it fails to produce the desired results. Women who undergo in vitro can also be damaged psychologically when the procedure does not work. If a woman is pursuing in vitro because she feels unfulfilled as a woman, failing to conceive despite advanced technology will only send her deeper into depression. Both partners pursuing a pregnancy via reproductive technologies can become obsessed with their goal, indulging in what has been characterized as "addictive, gambling-type behavior" (Hopkins qtd. In Neumann "Should health" 1216).

Many exposés of reproductive technology have been written by feminist critics. Authors such as Gena Corea, Renate Duelli Klein, Helen B. Holmes, Betty B. Hoskins, Christine Overall, and Robyn Rowland are only a few of the many prolific writers who have explored this topic. They have backgrounds in psychology, sociology, medicine, biology, philosophy, women's studies, political science, journalism, literature, and the law. From this multiplicity of perspectives, they have done an excellent job of exploring the ethical, legal, social, physical, and psychological repercussions of applying medical technology to birth, and specifically to women's bodies. They are for the most part, however, preaching to the already converted—or at least to a very narrow audience of well-educated and critical readers. Few of these feminist critics use case histories themselves when they explore new approaches to birth. Instead, their essays are very academic, very analytical. [5]

Where they are put to use, case histories can be extremely powerful rhetorical tools. Because they are mini biographies, part fiction, part reality, they allow us to peer into the personal and private lives of those whose stories they reenact. Case histories are very emotional texts, arousing our passions and stirring our sympathies; they appeal to the voyeur in all of us. We identify with the women whose stories we become privy to, thinking, "there but for the grace of God go I" or "maybe I can do what she has done."

Because the gynecological case history has such a strong appeal to the popular audience, an exploration of its conception in nineteenth-century medical texts and its subsequent appropriation by the popular media should help that audience to see how powerful it can be. Most of us are consumers of some form of popular media: lifestyles publications, commentary journals, news magazines and papers, and literature. Since this type of case history is becoming more and more influential in the popularization of the latest "advances" in reproductive technologies, it is wise to analyze its rhetoric to determine how it operates on our unconscious belief systems to bring us messages about these technologies.

In his 1985 essay, "The Bounds of Thinkable Thought," Noam Chomsky says, "there can be no more urgent task than to come to understand the mechanisms and practices of indoctrination" (31). He explains that in a democracy the boundaries are carefully—and subtly—drawn around the acceptable positions and opinions on certain topics, so as to rule out the possibility of challenging an idea or practice wholesale. In Chomsky's words, these mechanisms are "overwhelmingly effective in establishing a framework of thinkable thought" (31).

Chomsky's definition of indoctrination suggests that rhetorical analysis must look beyond this framework of thinkable thought to discover that which has been excluded by the boundaries. Kenneth Burke adds a moral imperative to this sort of analysis: "the rhetorician and the moralist become one at that point where the attempt is made to reveal the undetected presence of . . . an identification" (*Rhetoric* 26). Burke is speaking of the identification between science and imperialist-militaristic concerns; in the case history, the work of the rhetorician/moralist is to look for the hidden connections between science and capitalistic concerns. Selling women and their partners on reproductive technology means that hundreds of thousands of dollars will be infused into the medical economy. In addition, this technology allows doctors to perform a type of quality control over the end product. Fertility clinics of the future can compete not only for the high birth rates but also for the perfection of the child, just as some sperm banks already lay claim to having sperm encoded with superior genetic characteristics.[6]

Why look at the case history to find this connection between science and capitalistic concerns? As a sub-genre the case history has become daily fare in our popular media. Burke tells us: "we must think of rhetoric not in terms of some one particular address, but as a general *body of identifications* that owe their convincingness much more to trivial repetition and dull daily reënforcement than to exceptional rhetorical skill" (26). Our popular media is engaged in drafting just such a "body of identifications," a body that is already hard at work indoctrinating the readership of these publications. The relative strength or weakness of the rhetorical skills being exercised is less a factor than the sheer repetition of the thing. The case history, thanks to its sheer ubiquitousness, is one of the most influential tools of the reproductive industry.

Social psychologist Robyn Rowland writes that "[p]art of the strategy of social control which powerful groups use is the construction of a language which creates a 'softening up phase', [sic] language which prepares people for technologies which would otherwise be unacceptable" (230). "Reprospeak" (231), her term for this language, includes seemingly innocuous expressions like "surrogate mother." This term is used to describe a woman who agrees to gestate a child for a couple willing to pay certain fees for the service. The embryo will either be created by artificially inseminating the woman with the man's sperm, or it will be created in vitro with the egg and sperm of the contracting couple and then implanted into the uterus of the gestating woman. The word surrogate implies that the woman who gestates the fetus is the substitute mother of the child she carries even though she often "supplies" her own egg for the fetus and is as much a mother as she possibly can be. The term "surrogate mother" now has its own entry in the dictionary. *Webster's* defines it as "a woman who helps a couple to have a child by carrying to term an embryo conceived by the couple and transferred to her uterus; gestational carrier" (1345). The fact that the editors of the dictionary have adopted a definition implying the most remote relationship possible between mother and fetus shows how powerfully the term euphemizes this relationship.

Rowland explains that the end result of the linguistic promotion of technology is that while one woman (the infertile wife) is depicted as defective and inefficient, the other (the contract mother) is portrayed as capable of detaching herself from her baby. These characterizations pave the way for the objectification and control of women's bodies and the commodification and sale of their children.

In his discussion of the representative anecdote, Burke explains how the selection of terminology operates: "Men seek for vocabularies that will be faithful *reflections* of reality. To this end, they must develop vocabularies that are *selections* of reality. And any selection of reality must, in certain circumstances, function as a *deflection* of reality" (*Grammar* 59). Thus, we can see how the term "surrogate" emphasizes only a portion of the gestating woman's role in the creation of new life—her legal arrangement with the people who have contracted for her services. The result is that the term deflects reality by fixing its scope too narrowly. Because of the problematic nature of the expression "surrogate mother," I will instead use "contractual motherhood" to describe this practice and "contract mother" or some variation of "the woman who acts as surrogate" to identify women playing this role.[7]

On a scale larger than individual terms, an analysis of gynecological case histories will demonstrate how a too-narrowly-selected representative anecdote can restrict our view of a specific technology. Burke warns that "'[i]f you don't select one [anecdote] that is representative in a good sense, it will function as representative in a bad sense'" (324). Exploring the less-than-representative-anecdote from a Burkean perspective will mean looking into its constituent parts by using the dramatistic theory expressed in Burke's pentad.

The pentad is a heuristic device that allows its user to consider the relationships among five elements of an event. These elements—act, agent, agency, scene, and purpose—are very similar to the questions a journalist answers when reporting an event, except that Burke is more interested in the dramatic interaction between given elements. The elements can be defined as follows: act is the action engaged in, physical or linguistic; agent is the actor who performs the act; agency is the means by which the act is performed; scene is the physical or rhetorical context for the act; and purpose is the motivation the agent has for performing the act. For example, the pentad can be used to examine how an agent or performer of an action responds within a given rhetorical context or scene. At the same time this influence can be reciprocal: the scene itself may also be shaped by the nature of the agent. How one defines the elements of an event can also shift. The narrator of a case history can be defined as the agent in one set of relationships or as the agency or tool of those who publish the narrative.

To understand the modern gynecological case history, this study will begin with its precursor in nineteenth-century gynecology textbooks. The practice of gynecology (from the Greek for woman and discourse) was by no means a new specialty for nineteenth-century doctors, but scientifically trained practitioners were renewing their interest. The first entry on the topic that appeared in the Encyclopedia Britannica, volume XI of the Ninth Edition (published in volumes, 1875-89) was quite brief: "that branch of medicine which concerns the pathology and treatment of affections peculiar to the female sex" (350). In contrast, the entry in the Eleventh edition is several pages long; it explains the history of the practice and identifies symptoms and treatments for various gynecological problems: "The papyrus of Ebers, which is one of the oldest known works on medicine and dates from 1550 B.C., contains references to diseases of women, and it is recorded that specialism in this branch was known amongst Egyptian medical practitioners" (Encyclopedia Britannica 11th ed. Vol. XII 764). The extensive entry in the Eleventh edition shows how much interest and knowledge had increased in just the 35-year period between entries.

In chapter two, "Gynecology Undercover(s)," this period of growth and change will be explored. The progenitor of the modern gynecological case history will be studied to see how it was used to introduce young medical students to the scientific tenets of gynecology, and to convince the new male practitioners and their clients that the practice of studying living women's intimate organs was appropriate. By helping to break taboos against the public discussion of subjects considered to be immodest, gynecological case histories changed social attitudes about medicine and propriety. Thus for chapter two, the medical text of modest nineteenth-century society forms the scene for the act of discussing gynecological conditions and situations through the agency of the case history. The medical doctor acts as the agent performing this act for the purpose of instructing his colleagues and persuading potential patients to seek out his services.

As a scientific text, the case history has evolved into the highly objective account of patients' illnesses we find in modern medical journals, but where it has been appropriated by popular texts, it has maintained its personal appeal, its folksy quality, and its ability to affect the sensibilities of the public reader. The print media, combined with the new reproductive technologies made possible by medical science, create a far different scene for the twentieth-century case history. This new setting has produced significant changes in the elements of act, agency, agent, and purpose. A whole new menu of gynecological experiences is now being discussed by a more diverse group of authors. These agents—no longer likely to be medical authorities—have different purposes for their representations of reproductive technologies. These purposes will be determined by the specific scenes in which the modern case histories appear: the lifestyles publication, the commentary journal, the daily and weekly news media, and the literary text.

On July 25, 1978, Louise Joy Brown was born by cesarean section in Oldham, England. With her birth, the era of modern reproductive technology was born, along with the modern gynecological case history. Little Louise was the world's first "test-tube" baby, created by mixing her mother's egg with her father's sperm in a laboratory petri dish (not a test-tube as many assume). This first successful in vitro fertilization experiment was conducted by Dr. Patrick Steptoe and physiologist Robert Edwards. The team later came to be known as the "fathers" of in vitro fertilization.

The story of Louise Brown and her parents is an appealing one. The couple longed for a biological child and Louise fulfilled that desire. Her middle name is a testimony to her parents' reaction to her birth. The print media reacted to the birth as well, giving birth itself to a new type of article discussing or profiling the results of reproductive technologies. A study of general interest magazines published in North America between 1977 and 1997 maps the evolution of this new sub-genre. The study, done on publications categorized as academic, business, commentary, health, lifestyles, news, science/technology, and sociology, shows a dramatic leap in coverage of medically assisted births from 1977 to 1978.

Figure 1. shows that in 1977 one article on the topic of assisted reproduction appeared in *Good Housekeeping*, a lifestyles publication. (See Figures 2. and 3. for a breakdown of the categories.) In 1978, 42 articles were published by magazines in all of the above categories. Of these articles, only three are not directly related to the birth of Louise Joy Brown.

Further study of the coverage of reproductive technology in general interest magazines shows that this coverage appears to be driven by the case history, and for the most part, specifically by the controversial and sensational case history. Figure 1., which records a total of 877 publications in all eight categories, shows the 1978 leap mentioned above, then a decline to 20 articles in 1979. In 1980, "Elizabeth Kane," the first "legal" contractual mother gave birth and cooperated in a publicity campaign to make contractual motherhood more socially acceptable. At the same time, Robert Graham set up shop in Escondito, California. His "Repository for Germinal Choice" advertised itself as a sperm bank specializing in the sperm of Nobel Prize winners. These two events provoked quite a textual reaction. Magazine coverage increased to 29 articles in 1980.

From 1981 to 1986, the coverage evened out to an average of 18 articles per year. In 1987 total articles rose to 50, then shot to a high of 88 in 1988, followed by 76 in 1989. What happened? In 1986 Mary Beth Whitehead began the most publicized custody battle of the decade (perhaps the century) when she sued William Stern for custody of the baby girl she had contracted to carry for him and his wife. "Baby M" stories flooded the media until well after the New Jersey Supreme Court settled the case in 1988. In 1987, 26 articles were printed about the Baby M case, 15 were printed in 1988, and nine appeared in 1989.

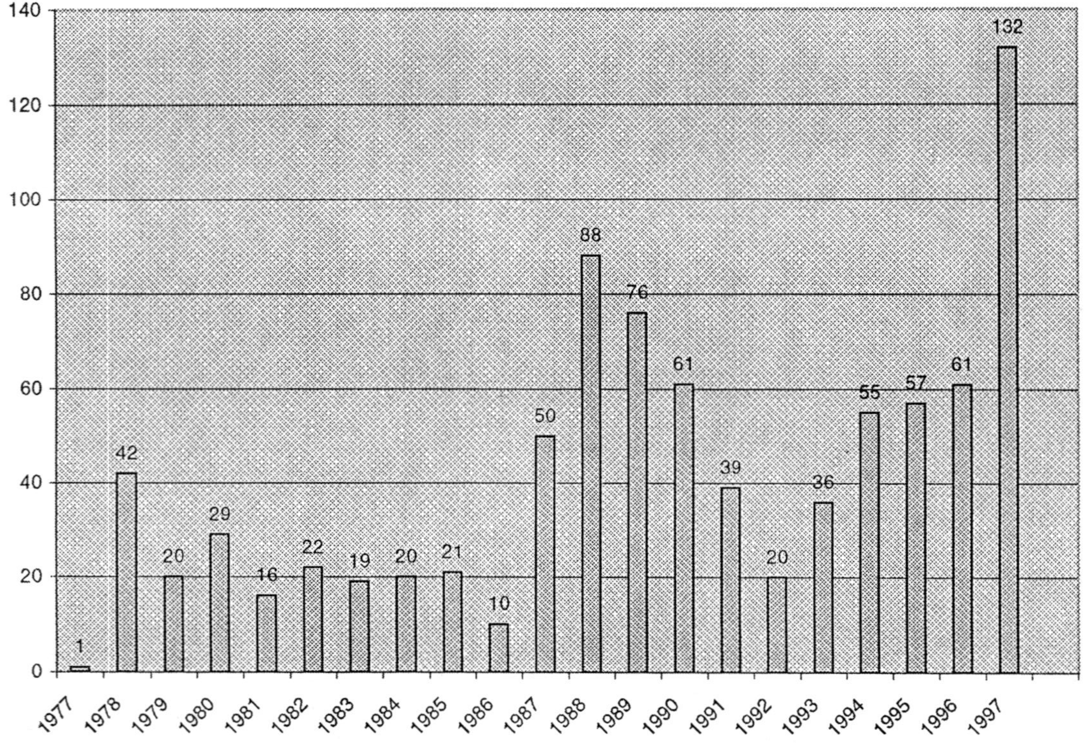

Fig. 1. Reproductive Technology Articles: Total of 877 in All Categories

The case also provoked intense discussion of the practice of what had come to be known as "surrogacy," with 14 articles published on the general topic in 1987, 29 articles appearing in 1988, and 18 printed in 1989.

By 1990, medical innovations had stimulated new controversies. Anna Johnson made the nation aware of "gestational surrogacy" by suing for custody of the baby boy she claimed to have bonded with. The judge ruled her a "genetic stranger" and awarded custody to the couple who had provided the egg and sperm. By 1992, overall magazine coverage had evened out again, this time to 20 articles. Then in October of 1993, Dr. Jerry Hall successfully cloned an embryo in his laboratory, and the media reacted with 36 articles that year and 55 the following. However, nothing has provoked discussion as much as two events that took place in 1997. First, scientists in Scotland cloned an adult lamb and second, an Iowa woman named Bobby McCaughey gave birth to surviving septuplets. Articles in four of the publication types—news, commentary, science and technology, and socio/environmental reached all-time highs; the total for all categories was 132 articles.

The lifestyle category, comprised mainly of women's service and fashion magazines, includes parenting magazines and general interest selections such as *People Weekly*, *The New Yorker*, *Reader's Digest*, and *TV Guide*. This type of publication focuses on humor, fiction, entertainment, improving personal lifestyles, and profiles of both the famous and the ordinary. Because reproductive technologies are practiced on women, chapter three, "Gynecology at the Check-out Stand," will focus only on the women's magazines in this grouping. In this setting, the author of the case history is often the woman who is the recipient of reproductive technology. She tells her story for a variety of reasons: to announce and authenticate her attainment of motherhood; to inform other women about the services available to them; to validate her feelings about what she has done—or has had done to her; to persuade others that her actions are acceptable; and on rare occasions, to warn other women of the potential harmful effects of reproductive technologies. Because the women's magazine has an agenda of its own—promoting motherhood—both the purpose of the case history and its agency are altered when it is adopted for this medium. The case history is presented as a fairy-tale quest for motherhood with a happy ending. The women's magazines' adoption of miracle metaphors to

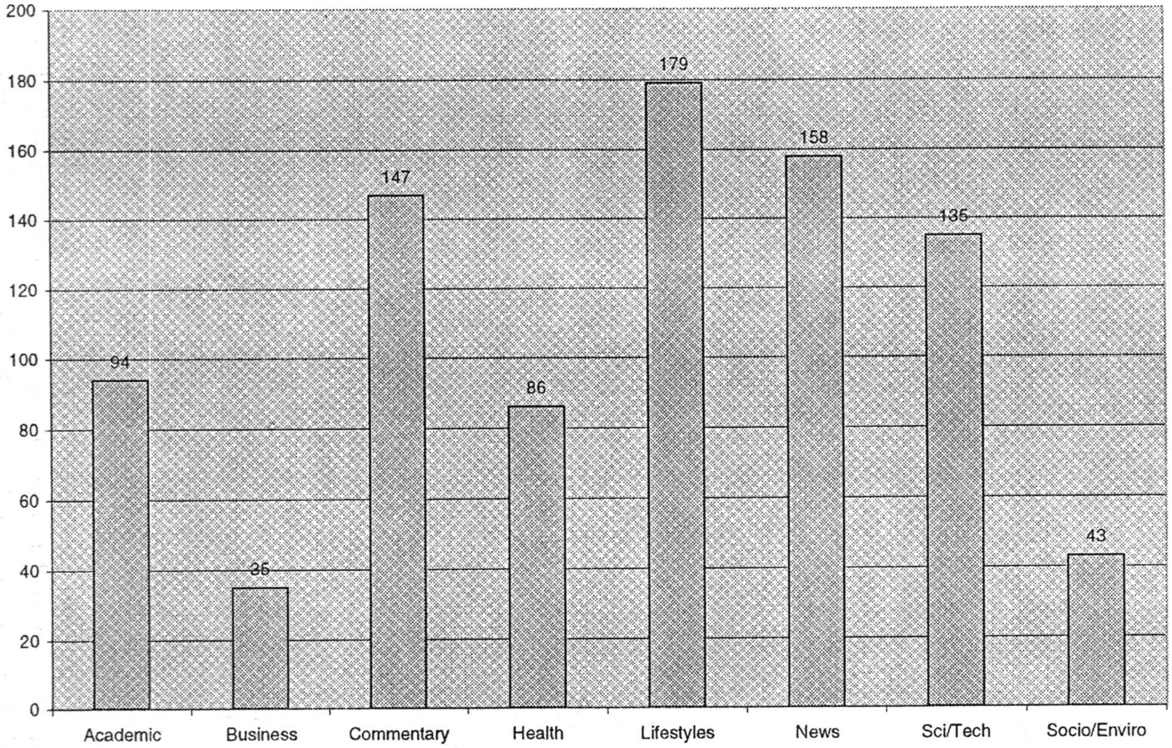

Fig. 2. Articles by Periodical Category: Total Articles 1977-1997

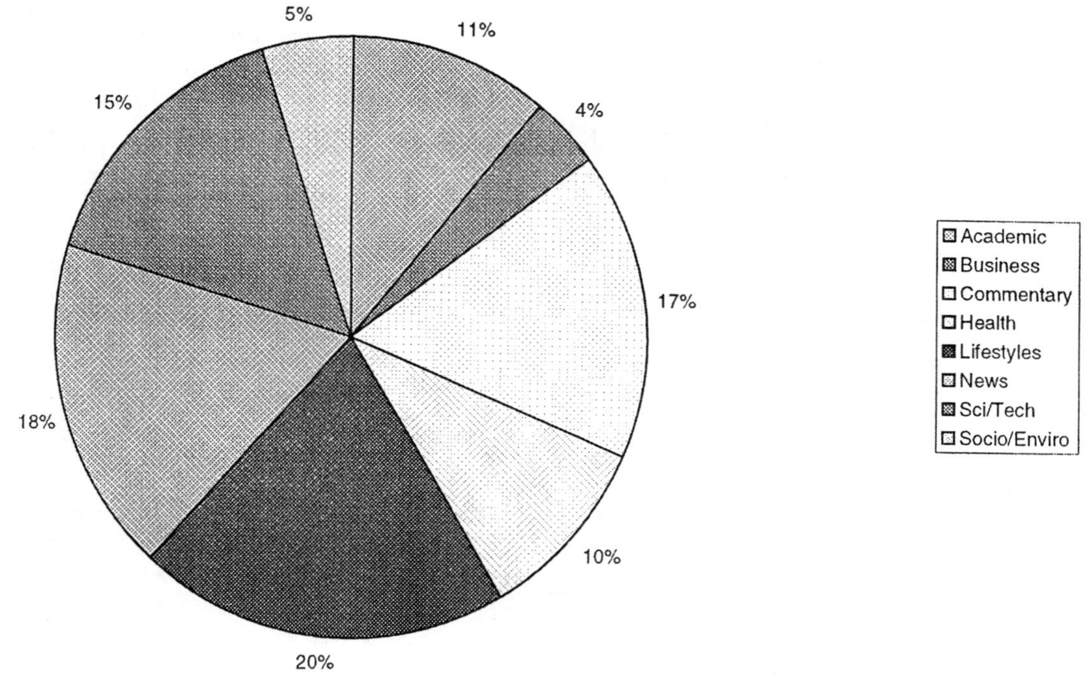

Fig. 3. Percentage of Total Articles by Category

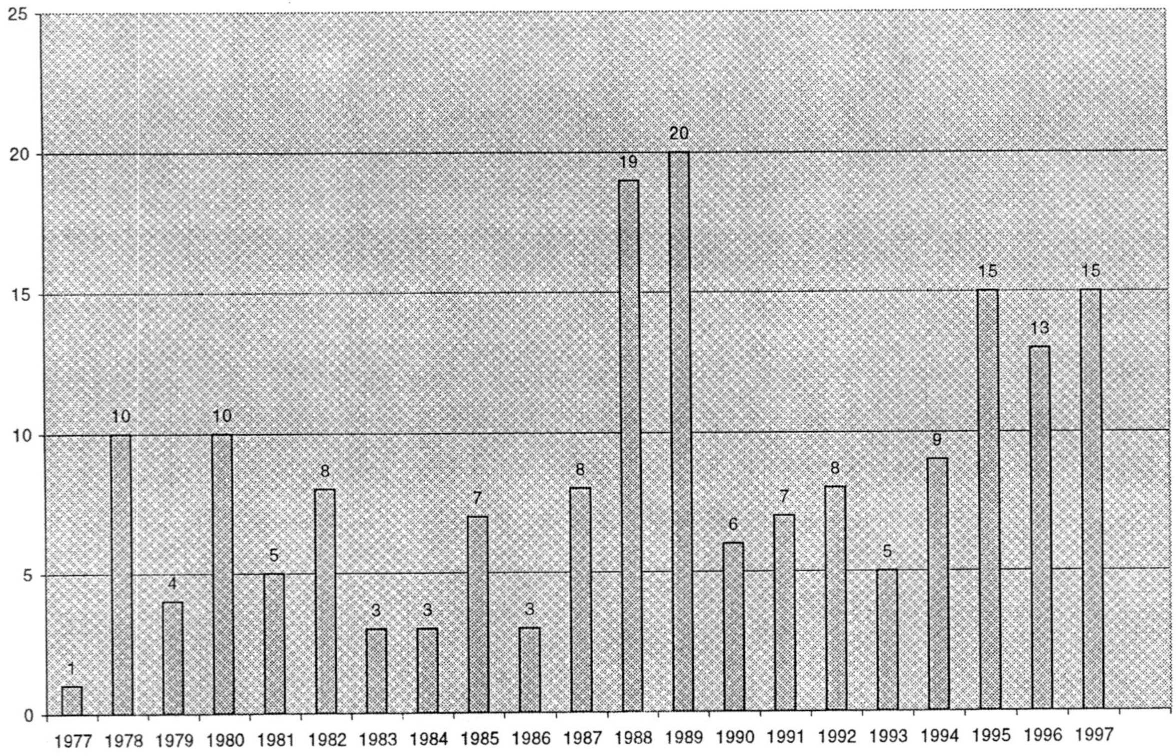

Fig. 4. Lifestyles Articles: Total of 179 Articles 1977-1997

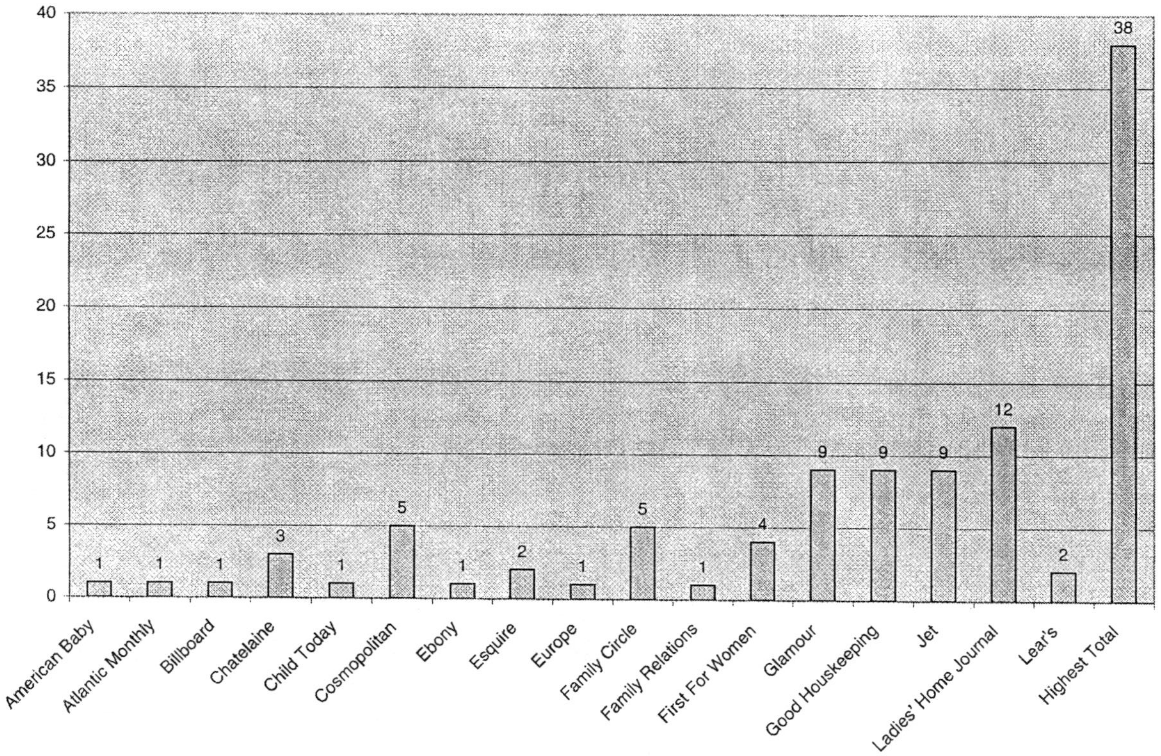

Fig. 5a. Articles in Lifestyles Magazines

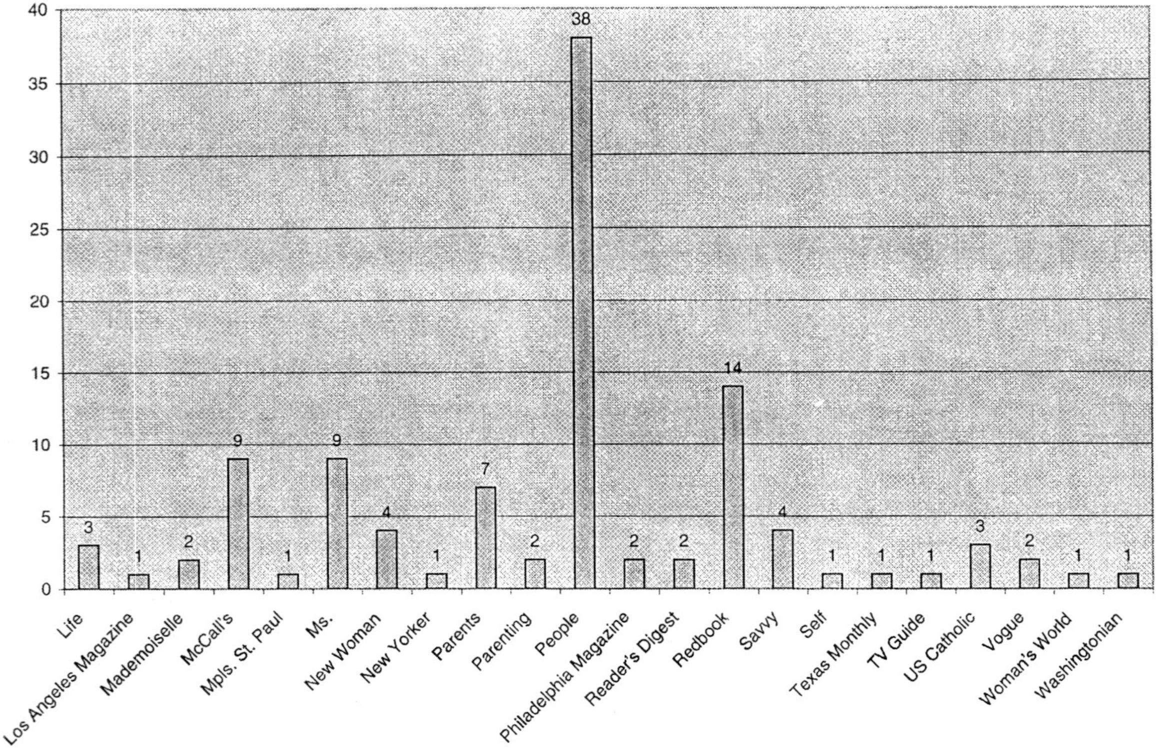

Fig. 5b. Articles in Lifestyles Magazines

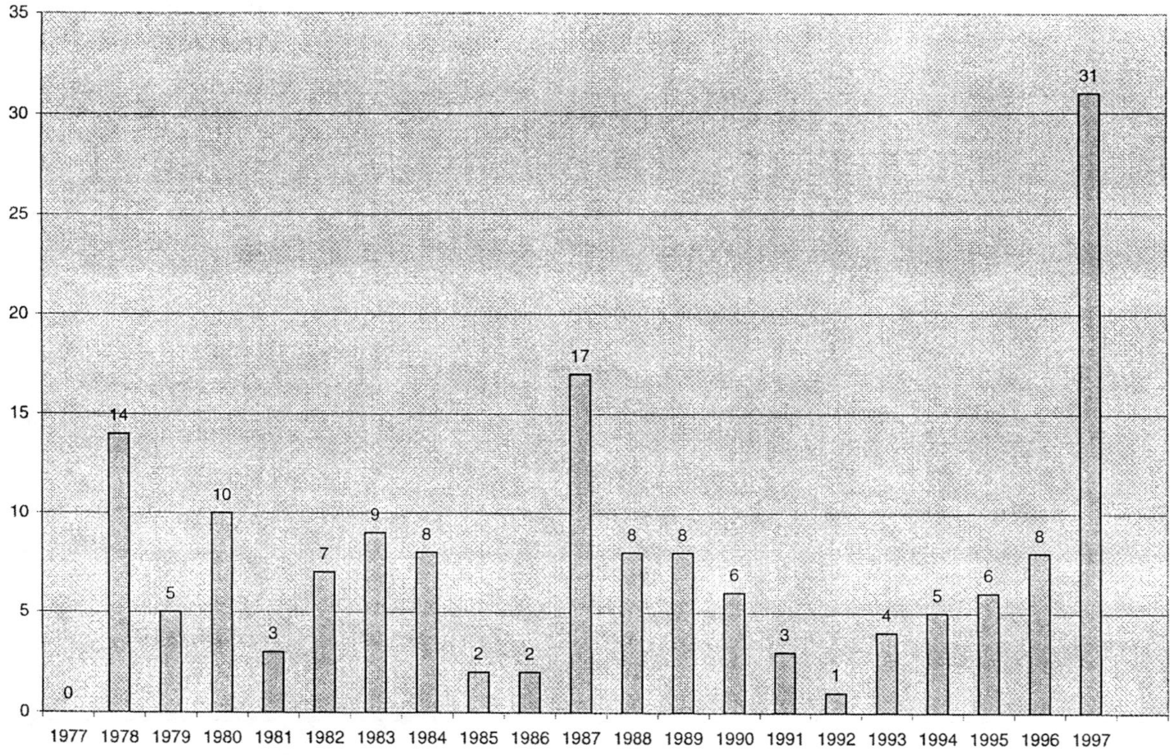

Fig. 6. News Articles: Total of 158 Articles 1977-1997

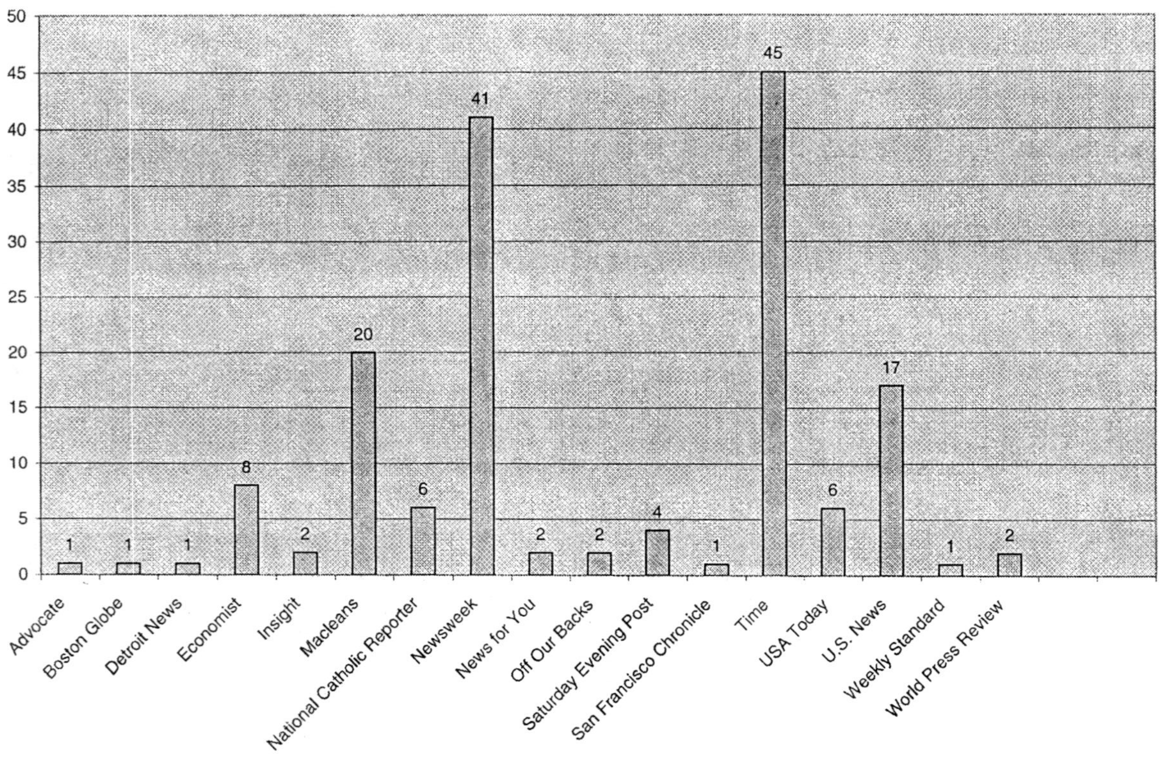

Fig. 7. Articles in News Magazines

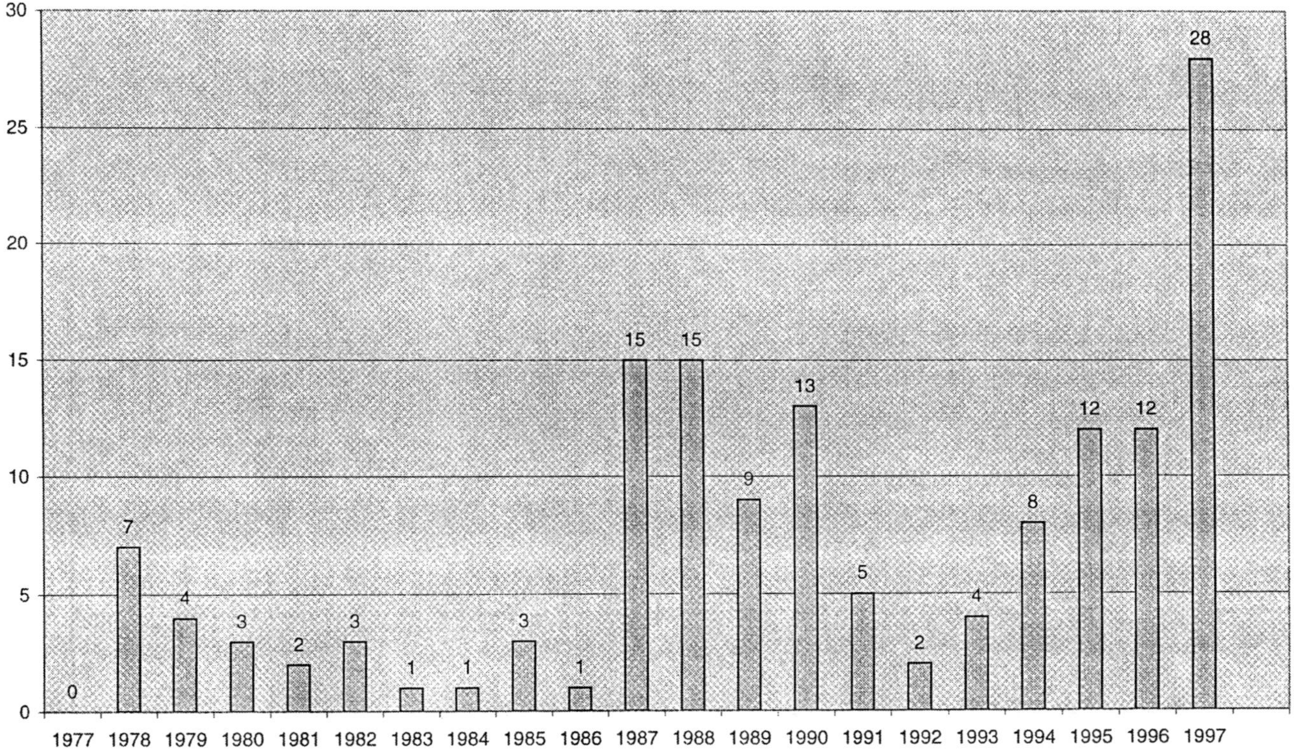

Fig. 8. Commentary Articles: Total of 147 Articles 1977-1997

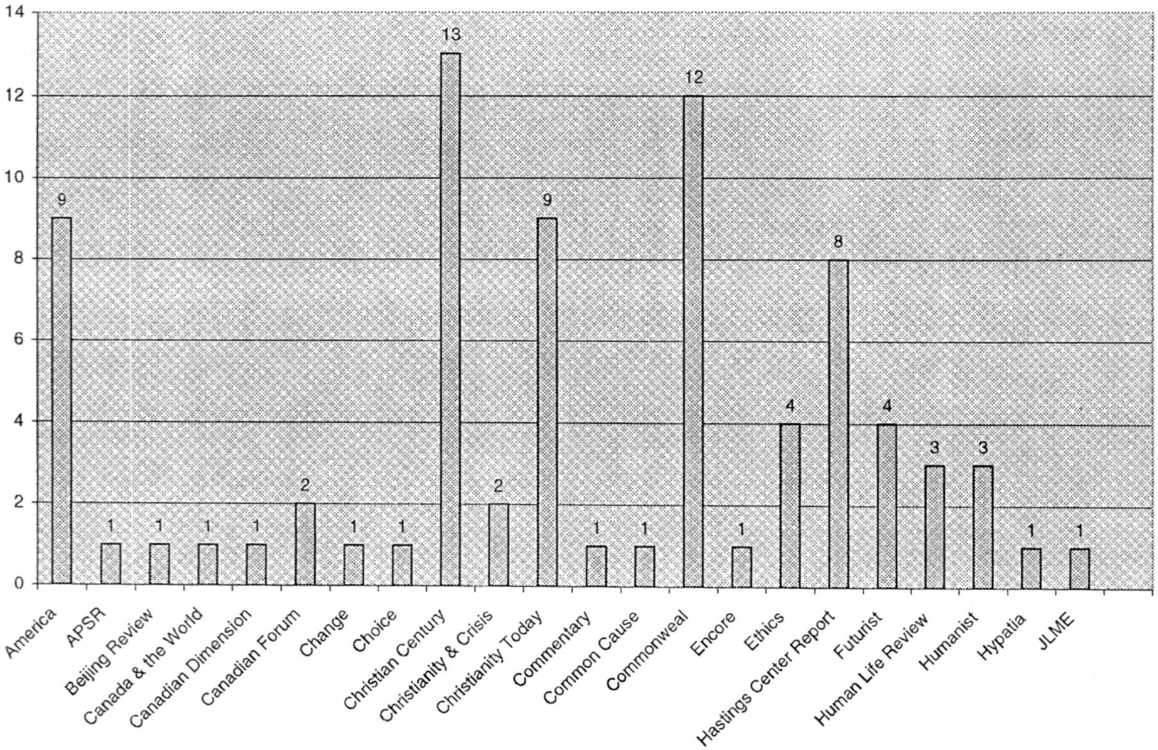

Fig. 9a. Articles in Commentary Journals

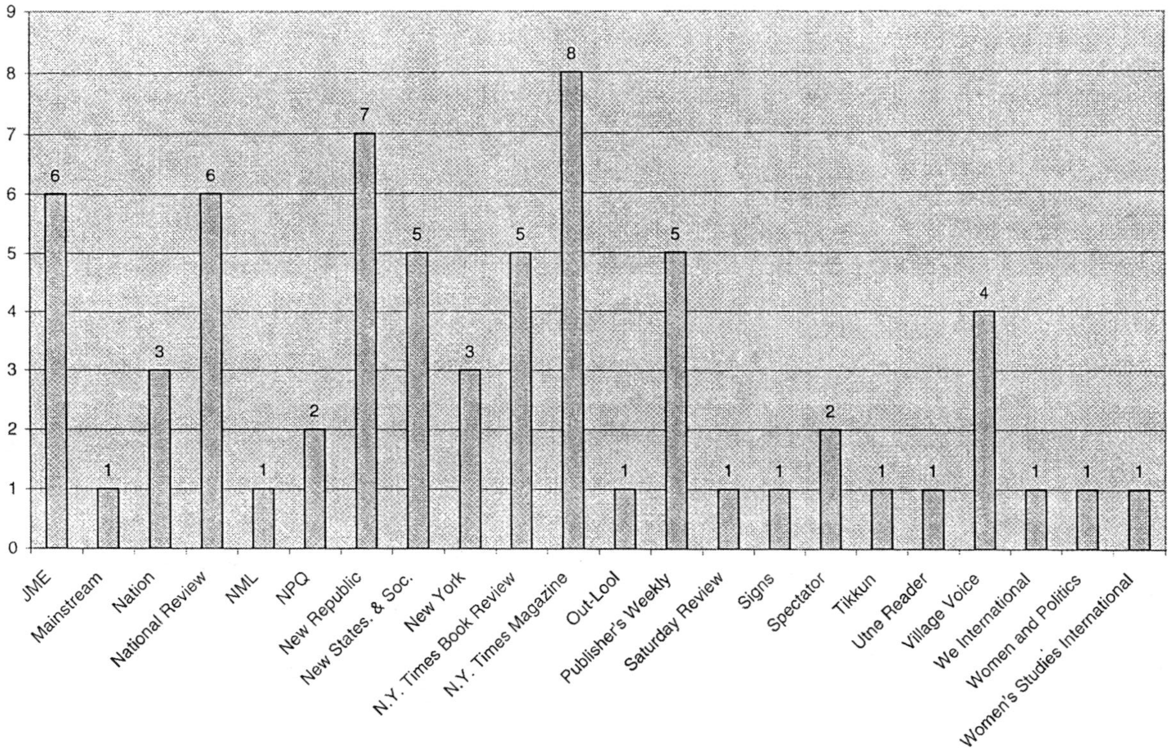

Fig. 9b. Articles in Commentary Journals

characterize technologically assisted birth allows the new technologies and their administrators to be aligned with God and his purposes. God's endorsement makes a critical discussion of these practices difficult, if not impossible.

In contrast to the happy endings presented by the lifestyles publications, a scene change to the commentary journal shows coverage that seems to be based almost entirely on reacting to controversial cases. Chapter four, "Gynecology on the Coffee Table," will look at how these publications represent the latest advances in reproductive technology. The commentary-style publications show a pattern of coverage on reproductive issues almost identical to the pattern created by the magazine industry in general. Figure 8. illustrates the way in which the commentary magazines have reacted to the sensational events of the past seventeen years, most notably the birth of Louise Joy Brown, the Baby M custody fight, and the debate over cloning. Figures 9a. and 9b. show by the breakdown of magazines within the commentary category that the Christian journals far outpace all of the others in their attention to the topic. *Christian Century*, *Commonweal*, *Christianity Today*, and *America*, together make up 29% of the total commentary coverage of 147 articles.

The authors of these commentary pieces differ a great deal from the authors of the articles in the lifestyles magazines. Their primary focus is on moral and ethical issues and their purpose is to open debate by presenting a strongly felt and argued position. The commentator, like the nineteenth-century doctor, is usually discussing someone else's experience. He/she uses the case as a springboard for the discussion of issues and ideals close to his/her heart: religious beliefs for some and feminist ideals for others. Many of the discussions within the pages of these journals are critical of the new technologies; however, though they respond to the issues raised by the cases, and pose some very serious moral and ethical questions, their coverage tends to end when the controversy fades or is upstaged by yet another reproductive feat.

In chapter five, "Gynecology at the Breakfast Table," the scene switches to the daily and weekly news media. The journalist who reports on the gynecological case history to the public is primarily interested in stories that will inform and engage a wide general audience. The daily news cannot wait for the refinement that accompanies a revised text, so in the newspaper the case history may appear as a rather cursory presentation of an interesting or controversial event. Because the news attempts to achieve objectivity, the voices of authorities from a variety of disciplines will often populate the text, with the reporter playing the role of conductor rather than commentator. The news magazine's weekly schedule provides the opportunity for a more sustained discussion of controversial events, and a good opinion piece can rival its counterpart in the commentary journal.

This focus on reporting the news creates coverage of reproductive technology that is more evenly distributed over the twenty-one-year period than that of the other categories. The characteristic increases do occur in 1978 and 1987; however, the drop in attention we saw in other publication categories between 1981 and 1986 does not hold true for the news publications.

Chapter six, "Gynecology in Dystopia," will look at the literary case history as a sort of coda to the previous chapters. By focusing specifically on three works we will look at what happens when the elements of fantasy and critique are combined in a representation of reproductive technology that does not have to remain true to any specific facts. Instead, by virtue of their total authority over the text, the authors can send their readers powerfully crafted messages embedded within fictitious gynecological stories that may come closer to reality than the real-life stories reported in our popular media. All three authors take their roles as social critics very seriously. Aldous Huxley's *Brave New World*, Margaret Atwood's *The Handmaid's Tale*, and Sarah Bird's *The Mommy Club*, all present fabricated case histories in which the repercussions of reproductive technology and the attitudes that make it possible are paramount.

Tracing the genesis and evolution of the gynecological case history shows its remarkable adaptability. The case history is a powerful rhetorical tool and it derives some of that power from its ability to change its agency as new relationships are formed between scene, purpose, act, and agent. Since it is likely that reproductive technologies will be refined as we move into the twenty-first century, it is also probable that the case history will be refined along with them, adjusting itself to accommodate new technological options and to present these options in new venues. One thing is certain, the complex technologies we have crafted will require significant revision to Burke's "Definition of Man" to make it appropriate for the next century.

NOTES

1. Burke uses the masculine gender throughout his discussion, so when quoting from or speaking about Burke's definition, I shall use his terms to define all of humanity. In my subsequent discussion, I shall use the term man to refer only to the masculine half of the species.

I am sure that Burke intended his definition to include women; however, in the conclusion to this book the reader will find my revision of Burke's definition in which I have attempted to accommodate woman's childbearing function. At this time, I also make my apologies to those feminists who reject an essentialist definition of woman, as mine is based entirely on our ability to reproduce.

2. The following list defines for the reader some of the reproductive technologies that are currently in use.

- AIH is artificial insemination using the "husband's" sperm.
- AID is artificial insemination using a donor's sperm.
- AIM combines the donor's sperm with the "husband's" so that the couple can hold on to the hope that the child is genetically related to its social father.
- Egg donation combines the use of a donated egg with in vitro fertilization so that a woman can carry a fetus not genetically related to her either because she intends to function as the child's gestational and social mother, or because she intends to function solely as the child's gestational mother while the woman who supplied the gamete will function as the child's social mother.
- Embryo flushing is a procedure in which the fertilized egg is "washed" out of one woman's uterus so it can be placed in another's.
- Fetal reduction is the euphemism for the practice of aborting selected fetuses when multiple pregnancies occur after superovulation or multiple implantation with in vitro.
- "Gestational" surrogacy is surrogacy ala Anna Johnson, in which the zygote, created from the egg and sperm of the contracting couple, is placed into the uterus of another woman who agrees to allow them the use of her body for gestation.
- GIFT is gamete intra-fallopian tube transfer. The egg and sperm are placed into the fallopian tube, allowing them to fertilize in the tube and giving them a better chance of implanting in the uterus.

- ICSI is intracytoplasmic sperm injection. Sperm that are incapable of fertilizing an egg on their own because of defect are forced beyond the egg's natural barrier to fertilize the egg.
- IVF "traditional" is old-hat now. The women's eggs are removed and inseminated, then replaced in her uterus.
- Sperm and embryo banking make use of freezing technique to preserve genetic materials in various stages of fertilization.

3. See note two for definitions of these two types of surrogacy.

4. The name Elizabeth Kane was a pseudonym used to protect her from publicity.

5. Linda Williams, Ellen Messer and Kathryne May are notable exceptions. Williams collected and used the stories of women who have undergone in vitro technologies to make her case that this "service" exacts much too high a price physically, emotionally, and psychologically from those it purports to help. Messer and May have collected accounts of abortions performed before Roe v. Wade made the procedure legal. Both texts make good use of the personal and emotional accounts of the women who helped to write them by sharing their stories.

6. The "Repository for Germinal Choice" in Escondito, California was established to house the sperm of Nobel Prize winners. It now also accepts sperm from men with extremely high IQs. Customers can leaf through profiles of the donors that include information about artistic and athletic ability, physical characteristics and religious affiliations. Robert Graham, the director, swears that sperm from his bank "breeds true." In other words, he believes that it is genetically stronger than the woman's egg and will dominate the child's characteristics (Lowry 12).

7. The term "contract mother" is not mine. I have borrowed it from feminist commentator Katha Pollitt who uses it in her discussion of the Baby M case printed in *The Nation*.

CHAPTER TWO

Gynecology Undercover(s)

> Obstetrics is that part of the science and art of medicine relating to the function of reproduction . . . . The obstetrician should not be a "midwife," caring only for actual births—his duty is to treat all the diseases and accidents that have to do with the reproductive function (xiii).
>
> Joseph B. De Lee M.D.
> *The Principles and Practice of Obstetrics*, 1936

The nineteenth-century gynecologist was an "undercover" practitioner. Doctor and patient alike were beset with moral qualms about the propriety of the practice. Because of these concerns, the doctor performed procedures on his blushing patients by feel—literally under the covers. To legitimize the increased male involvement in midwifery, a rhetoric had to be developed that would help the practitioner to talk with his peers and patients about very intimate concerns. A study of this rhetoric will show how the case history emerged as a tool for accomplishing the dual goals of instructing the doctor in his practice and selling the patient on his services. The modern gynecological case history has its beginnings here, in its nineteenth-century prototype.

> A distressing fear of the event of parturition, sometimes takes possession of pregnant women as the dreaded time approaches. Such should be taught reliance on the protection of *Providence.* If however this dread be attended with increased heat, a white scurf [encrustation] on the tongue, quick pulse, and especially if there be a fixed pain in the belly. . . it requires blood-letting, and frequently a repetition of it with gentle purges. (Jennings qtd. in Speert 37)

The above quote from an 1808 "Ladies' Companion" gives some idea of the state of obstetrical practice in the early nineteenth century. For at least the first quarter of the century, most births were attended by female midwives who rarely intervened in the birth process. Male practitioners were called in when relying on "Providence" proved unsuccessful, and "heroic medicine"—measures such as purges, blistering, emetics, and bloodletting—was deemed necessary (Edwards and Waldorf 150). By the end of the century, most of the major technologies that characterize basic twentieth-century gynecological practice had been developed. Male obstetricians were in control in the birthing room and intervention had become the norm rather than the exception. The case history was an integral part of these changes, serving as a means of transmitting personal experience from doctor to doctor, and from doctor to student. The case history was especially valuable to the male student who, unlike the midwife, began his studies with no personal experience on which to build his knowledge. In addition to its pedagogical function, the case history contributed to changing attitudes about male doctors treating female patients for the most intimate of "complaints." Doctors who wrote case histories were breaking taboos against speaking of these intimate subjects. The case history provided a safe forum for observing the female body in childbirth; it served a voyeuristic function that set the stage linguistically for the subsequent use of living patients to train students of obstetrics.

To understand the role the case history played, we must remind ourselves of the state of medical practice in the nineteenth century, and specifically, what was beginning to be referred to as "the science and art of obstetrics."[1] Most of the medical procedures and tools we take for granted in the late twentieth century were not available to the medical profession in the early nineteenth. Anesthesia and antisepsis had not been discovered yet. Major surgery was dangerous and performed only when there were no other options. Multiple approaches to healing abounded—some effective and some quite dangerous. The latter motivated prominent, European-trained doctors to argue for scientific training over other approaches. As early as 1765, doctors in Philadelphia and New York were advocating for systematic scientific training at medical colleges. Such training included "anatomy, material medicine, botany, chemistry, and clinical experience (Scholten 146). By 1807, five American schools offered courses in midwifery.

Despite the medical profession's growing interest in childbirth, for the first part of the nineteenth century most women were still attended by female midwives, in their own homes, and with their female relatives and close friends in attendance. Births remained a female-directed event even after women began to make use of the tools and drugs being offered by male practitioners (Scholten 150). As male practitioners gained ground, however, the open nature of the birthing room changed and control switched into the medically trained doctor's hands. The reasons for this change are complex. Industrialization brought many changes for women by "reshap[ing] the contours of domestic labor and thus . . . erod[ing] the stability of households" (Kerber 7). Scriptural reinterpretation implied that suffering in childbirth was not a biblical requirement, so religious attitudes towards women's suffering began to change (Scholten 147). With the newly industrialized economy adopting many of their traditional household functions, middle- and upper-class women organized physiological societies and became active in the nineteenth-century health reform movement (Morantz "Making Women Modern" 348). The movement was characterized by the belief that good health was not only a possibility, but also a personal responsibility. Reformers advised on healthy diets, counseled against restrictive dress like the corset, and advocated that women be educated in physiology so they could take on the task of caring for their family's health (348-350).

Women's involvement in health reform reflects changes in their roles brought on by a social and political evolution that had been taking place in America since the Revolutionary war. Historian Linda Kerber describes the political transformation: "A restrained, deferential democracy characteristic of American colonial loyalties gradually gave way to an aggressive, egalitarian, modern participatory democracy" (7). Egalitarian philosophy was adopted by women reformers who added new definitions to their traditional roles. The characteristics of the "cult of of true womanhood" identified by Barbara Welter as "purity, piety, domesticity, and submission" (103-113) were traditionally identified with women's work in the home. Reformers argued that the woman's sphere extended to the public and political. The "Republican Mother" (Kerber 7) was still playing the role of family caretaker even when she advocated for public health reform; just as the woman who argued for entrance into medical school was fulfilling her potential as nurturer.

A corollary of the change in attitude towards women's health and suffering was that doctors began to believe that the birth process was inherently flawed. They devoted themselves to improving on nature and relieving women of the suffering occasioned by pregnancy and childbirth (Scholten 147). This pathological view of pregnancy is fully worked out by Dr. Joseph B. De Lee in the 1936 edition of his popular gynecology textbook.

> Can a function so perilous that, in spite of the best care, it kills thousands of women every year, that leaves at least a quarter of the women more or less invalided, and a majority with permanent anatomic changes of structure, that is always attended by severe pain and tearing of tissues, and that kills 3 to 5 per cent. [sic] of children—can such a function be called normal? (xiv).

In response to this new mission of improving on the birth process, doctors refined crude tools such as the forceps, which had been invented by the Chamberlen family in the seventeenth century, and brought powerful drugs into the birthing room. Where midwives had traditionally used teas to ease labor, doctors tried ergot, ether, and chloroform (Edwards and Waldorf 150; Walzer Leavitt "Birthing" 175; Morantz "Making Women Modern" 351). These drugs, combined with better tools, allowed male practitioners to offer a good deal of relief to laboring women. They could both speed up and numb the process (though this was often done to the woman's or newborn's detriment). It should be noted that at the same time that the male practitioner rose in prominence by virtue of his access to scientific knowledge, the female midwife was denied such access and squeezed out of the profession. The result was that women lost control of a process that had for centuries been female-dominated (Scholten 148).

Birthing women themselves contributed to this change by seeking out the services offered by the scientifically-trained doctor. They did, in fact, have a "distressing fear of the event of parturition"—with good reason—and they did not want to leave their fates in the hands of Providence. Several factors contributed to high mortality rates for both women and their babies. Before the discovery of bacteria, infection was easily spread by both midwives and male practitioners. Without both antisepsis and anesthesia, little could be done for women with difficult labors. Babies often had to be removed with crude hooks and crotchets to save the mother's life (Scholten 146). Vesico-vaginal fistulas—tears in the vaginal wall and bladder—often caused by the inept and unnecessary use of forceps, would leave women as life-long invalids (Edwards and Waldorf 104). Additionally, fashion and lifestyle contributed to problems with labor and delivery. The corset, worn by most middle- and upper-class women, compressed the pelvic area, making delivery difficult if not impossible in some cases (Morantz "Making Women Modern" 349). With the advent of industrialization, lower class women worked long hours in factories and lived in crowded and unsanitary urban ghettos (349), while middle-and upper-class women languished at home. Working women were often exhausted by their work schedules and home responsibilities. Doctors attending to idle middle- and upper-class women warned them away from exercise and education. The confined and inactive lives that resulted led to chronic ailments (Edwards and Waldorf 152), confirming the medical view that "civilized" women were inherently flawed.[2]

For these reasons, birth could be a dangerous and painful experience, and any tool or procedure that promised to make it safer was welcomed by those who were afraid of potential problems in delivery. However, social disapproval of male birth attendants was high, and medical students were trained to use instruments only with illustrations and mannequins. The case history helped to fill in some of the gaps by providing a discussion about how doctors responded to difficult cases and improvised new procedures.

At the beginning of the nineteenth century, the United States had just three hospitals for the general public and five medical schools, where, though lectures in midwifery were offered, they were not required for a medical degree (Speert 37, 73-75). Those who could afford to travel studied in England, Scotland, or France (Cutter and Viets 145). When they returned, many of these men set up lecture series, often from their homes, for both midwives and new doctors. For aspiring doctors who could not afford to travel to Europe, or the tuition at an American school, lectures and apprenticeships were the only available methods of training. This training was often inadequate as anyone could announce lectures or declare himself an instructor and accept apprentices (72). As late as 1855, students were not provided with clinical experience and it was only in the last two decades of the century that schools began to require students to attend cases and participate in internship programs (76). Before these programs were instituted, the case history was often the only way in which medical students could gain an understanding of the practical problems they would encounter once they had finished their studies.

Perhaps the most prominent medical lecturer of the late eighteenth century was Dr. William Shippen, Jr. of Philadelphia. His training shows the common pattern for those who could afford to be well-educated in their profession. He began his medical training at the College of New Jersey (Princeton), apprenticed for three years with his father, Dr. William Shippen, and then went to Europe to study in Edinburgh (Cutter and Viets 147). In January of 1765, he announced a course of lectures on midwifery. The announcement reveals the growing distrust the medically trained doctor held toward the midwives who had attended births since the establishment of the American colonies:

> Dr. Shippen, Jr. having been lately called to the assistance of a number of women in the country, in difficult labors, most of which was made so by the unskillful old women about them, the poor women having suffered extremely, and their innocent little ones being entirely destroyed, whose lives might have been easily saved by proper management, and being informed of several desperate cases in the different neighborhoods which had proved fatal to the mothers as to their infants, and were attended with the most painful circumstances too dismal to be related, he thought it his duty immediately to begin his intended courses in Midwifery, and has prepared a proper apparatus for that purpose, in order to instruct those women who have virtue enough to own their ignorance and apply for instructions, as well as those young gentlemen now engaged in the study of that useful and necessary branch of surgery, who are taking pains to qualify themselves to practice in different parts of the country with safety and advantage to their fellow citizens (qtd. in Cutter and Viets 149).

This very positive characterization of the young medical student indicates an early attempt by the medical profession to establish the primacy of the scientific approach to obstetrics and to overcome the public's objections to male midwifery. In fact, many midwives were quite adept at their profession and many male practitioners were both as unqualified and as dangerous as those midwives who were incompetent.

Regulations covering medical practitioners were not routinely established until the end of the nineteenth century, when the American Medical Association (AMA), founded in the 1840s by Dr. Nathan Smith Davis, finally succeeded in establishing boards of medical examiners in all of the states (Speert 77-78). Before such regulations were enacted almost anyone could establish a medical practice and treat patients in any manner he/she chose. Many of these approaches were not scientific, ranging from homeopathy and hydropathy to downright charlatanism. The experience of the general public was very mixed; some people were saved by doctors, but some were killed by their methods. This uncertainty about the skills of anyone proclaiming to be a doctor meant that there was widespread distrust of the profession in general, and the admission of male practitioners into the modest woman's bedchamber was highly suspect. In the woman's handbook and medical guide, the case history worked to convince women and their spouses that they were better off being treated by the scientifically-trained male doctor than the "quack" practitioner (anyone not scientifically trained), or the often incompetent and superstitious female midwife.

The problems obstetricians experienced in practicing midwifery are explained by Dr. Irving S. Cutter in his 1933 history of obstetrics. His interpretation reflects the profession's position on the male/female question:

> As may be understood, Shippen's efforts to create enthusiasm for midwifery were fraught with much discouragement. While medicine and surgery were dominant and under the immediate jurisdiction of trained *men*, midwifery was relegated for the most part to ignorant *women* who fostered the idea that it was improper and indelicate for a woman in labor to be attended by a male physician. (My emphasis 150)

Cutter's interpretation is questionable here, however, because "ignorant women" certainly were not the only ones who held the opinion that male midwifery was indelicate and even immoral. The attitude prevalent at the time is expressed by Samuel Gregory, whose 1848 pamphlet, "Man-Midwifery Exposed and Corrected," labeled man-midwifery as immoral. Gregory believed that its practice threatened the morality of both the male practitioner and his patient. "'[T]he unlimited intimacy between a numerous profession and the female population silently and effectually wears away female delicacy and professional morality, and tends, probably more than any other cause in existence, to undermine the foundations of public virtue'" (qtd. in Speert 18). Members of this new obstetric specialty were well aware of their patients' reluctance to expose themselves to male practitioners. Students were urged to act like gentlemen at all times, to convey intimate questions and information through other women present, and to delay examinations until the lights were dimmed and the birthing woman was in the middle of a contraction, if possible (Scholten 149). Husbands shared their wives' reluctance. Historian Catherine Scholten reports one American gentleman sending for a male midwife and then telling him that "'he would demolish him if he touched or looked at his wife'" (qtd. in Scholten 149).

At the same time that men were moving into the midwife's territory, women were seeking access to medical training. Their argumentative strategies included the propriety issue. Using the belief in women's moral superiority, they argued that male midwives compromised women's modesty. Elizabeth Blackwell, the first woman to receive a medical degree in the United States, labeled male-midwifery an "'unnatural and monstrous arrangement'" (qtd. in Morantz "The Connecting Link" 164). The goal of their argument was to gain access to medical training, but social attitudes about women's ability to learn the disciplines involved—languages, mathematics, chemistry—were difficult to overcome (Scholten 148). Nineteenth-century women did gain access to medical training, but the midwife did not fare so well. By the middle of the century, doctors had stopped offering lectures to midwives and had begun to focus their training manuals on their male medical students. The campaign to discredit the midwife was in full swing as doctors saw her lack of scientific training as a threat to their newly professionalized discipline and her practice as a threat to their incomes (Scholten 148; Kobrin 201).

Working against arguments of impropriety were the all too common problems caused by the female midwife's superstitious practices and lack of training. Speert characterizes the midwife as "untrained, ignorant, often illiterate, and superstitious" (11). He recounts some of their more colorful superstitious practices:

> Some granny-women in the Ozarks always carried with them coins stolen from the church in the belief that this money placed in the parturient's mattress would ease the pains of labor. Others hung an empty hornet's nest in the patient's attic. Still others placed an ax under the bed to make a difficult birth easier, but only after the edge was brought to razor sharpness, for a dull ax was likely to do more harm than good. (11)

This is the context in which the early case histories functioned. The main goals for the scientific practitioners of midwifery, as outlined above, were establishing public approval of the male accoucheur, and eliminating non-scientific approaches. The case history was to contribute to both of these goals by giving the obstetrician a forum in which to discuss medical cases and procedures without being considered improper. Gynecological case histories became a genre through which medical knowledge and ideology could be transmitted to the student, and later, in women's handbooks, to the patient herself.

The first case histories to appear in an American textbook can be found in Samuel Bard's *Compendium of the Theory and Practice of Midwifery*. Its publication in 1807 made it the first gynecology textbook to be written in America. Like Shippen, Bard studied first in America, apprenticed with his doctor father, and completed his studies in Edinburgh. His book was written after his retirement and included the wisdom he had gained from his thirty-three years in medical practice (Speert 74).

The first edition of the text is written for the midwife and reflects the same concern for overcoming her ignorance as Shippen's lecture announcement. Bard, however, includes untrained practitioners in his concern:

> Having frequently, in the course of my practice, and particularly since my residence in the country, had occasion to observe how much our midwives, and too many practitioners, who take on themselves the care of women in labour, stand in need of instruction, and how incapable most of such are, from deficiency of education, as well as from pecuniary considerations, to derive it from books of science and systems of midwifery, I have thought that a concise, cheap book, containing plain, but correct rules for their practice in natural labours, and for the relief of such complaints as frequently accompany

> pregnancy and labour, or which follow delivery, would, in the present state of this country, prove a useful work. (iii)

Because this first edition was written with the midwife in mind, Bard does not include case histories in any substantial number. He discusses problems in generalities, most likely relying on the experience the midwife would bring to her reading of the book to fill in the gaps. When editing the fourth edition, however, Bard had redefined the audience as medical students. This revision necessitated the addition of more scientific language and medical plates. Most important, Bard "illustrated the doctrines by a great number of cases, drawn from the best authorities, and particularly from the latest and most valuable periodical works" (B). Bard explains the utility of the case histories at the end of his 1819 introduction:

> This plan. . . I am persuaded, will be found particularly useful to the student, not only in explaining the doctrines and enforcing the best practice, . . . but as they [the cases] will be found to contain the soundest principles of general practice, and a variety of incidental occurrences, which (although they require particular management) cannot easily be interpreted into a systematic work. It is something like adding experience to theory, is a miniature representation of real practice; and if the cases are carefully studied, as I earnestly recommend them to be, will be found to imprint the principles of the art, and the rules of the practice, upon the mind of the student more permanently than any plan, simply didactic, can possibly do. (B)

The first edition of the book contains four case histories, two drawn from Bard's personal experience and two from accounts related to him by colleagues. All four concern the same problem—inverted uterus—a problem which was unusual and therefore must have required illustration. The fourth edition of the book contains 152 case histories; of these only four are drawn from Bard's personal experience. The rest are cited from 38 other doctors and four medical journals. The addition of 148 case histories and Bard's introductory comments make it clear that he believed the medical student would not have the same experiences to bring to his education as the midwife. The utility of the case history as a pedagogical tool seems clear; serving as a "miniature representation of real practice," these accounts were a substitute for attending living patients at a time when allowing medical students to do so would have caused a huge outcry in the populace.

If we compare the four case histories offered in Bard's first edition to those of the fourth edition, we can also see the influence of science at work. First, by simply quoting so many "experts," Bard has endeavored to increase his credibility. Of more interest is the difference in the way the case histories are reported. The following is Bard's personal account of a case of inverted uterus, printed in the first edition:

> A lady, very tall, after a labour rather tedious and severe, was at last, by one long and severe pain, delivered of her second child. On tying the navel-string, I observed it to be remarkably thick and very short, and on taking hold of it between my thumb and finger, (for I could not twist it around my finger) I perceived, as I thought, the placenta to be descending; not however, by successive pains, but by one continued uninterrupted descent, until it was thrown out of the vagina; and, to my very great astonishment, with it came the whole volume of the womb. It is not easy to express my feelings at that moment; still, however, I commanded so much presence of mind, as neither to lose my time nor alarm my patient. The placenta, which was already in part separated, was immediately detached, and my fingers being applied to the fundus of the womb, it was immediately and completely reverted, the hand and arm being introduced as high as the elbow, then slowly withdrawn. No flooding or other ill consequence ensued, and the patient speedily recovered. It was seven years before this lady became again pregnant; her labour was then natural and happy; she has since had a fourth child, and now enjoys good health. (175-176)

Bard's account is very personal and gives his reaction to the incident the same importance as the medical situation and the treatment. In fact, his purpose seems to be to explain how calmly he reacted to a situation he had never experienced before. This case is not one illustrating "the soundest principles of general practice," which is how Bard describes those included in the fourth edition. Instead it is, by comparison, an unscientific account of the doctor's personal experience.

In contrast, the case histories cited in the fourth edition sound much more scientific. The doctor is distanced from the experience through the use of an objective tone. We can compare a case taken from a Mr. Brandon Fry, who purports to have developed a cure for puerperal fever. Bard begins his account by explaining Fry's general method of treatment: bleeding, blistering, emetics (medicines that cause vomiting), antimonials (medicines incorporating a metallic element that have an emetic and diuretic effect), mercurials (medicines containing mercury, often used as an ointment), and deobstruents (diuretics). The case is presented chronologically, beginning with the twenty-first day, and includes significant events in the illness, along with the appropriate medical terms:

> 21st day. She has not been quite so well as usual for the last two or three days, and her pulse has been quick. . . . I find a circumscribed swelling and hardness, as of a large gland, in the right iliac region [the lower abdominal area], a little above Poupart's ligament. . . . I applied leeches to the pained part and gave her an emetic; and a blister was laid on as soon as the bleeding from the leeches had ceased.
>
> 22nd day. Patient much easier.
>
> 23d day. Leeches were again applied a little above the seat of the last blister, and were followed by another blister, laid upon the part to which they had been applied. An increase of relief was immediately perceived by the patient, and in a few days the soreness, swelling, and every other complaint were entirely gone. (362)

The focus here is on the etiology of the disease and the doctor's treatment of its symptoms, rather than the doctor's personal reaction to the patient and her suffering. In fact, when reading this case, one wonders about the doctor's emotions. Placed in the context of today's medical practices, the treatment sounds quite brutal. And in fact, the nineteenth-century health reform movement began largely in response to the type of "heroic therapy" described in this case. A nineteenth-century observer, William Corbett, wryly described such treatments as "one of the great discoveries which are made from time to time for the depopulation of the earth" (qtd. in Edwards and Waldorf 150). Presumably, the doctor acted to help the patient, but how did he react to the suffering his measures must have caused? The doctor's elimination of the personal and his medical focus illustrates the objective and scientific approach to healing that medicine was cultivating in the nineteenth century.

Bard's intention to write a plain book (one that would be understood by those untrained in science) also highlights early nineteenth-century attitudes towards writing about the subject of birth. Using purely scientific language would be far more acceptable, but Bard wants the book to be acceptable to the uneducated reader. He has to strike a balance between what will be understood and what will be considered proper by using "as few technical terms as was consistent with perspicuity and decency. . . (iv). Clearly, there were moral standards in operation that Bard had to consider when writing his book.

After Bard's use of the gynecological case history, the gynecology textbook remained a curious hybrid of scientific reasoning and anecdotal evidence. Its format and tone are far from standardized, and for some authors cases seem to have more in common with literature than with scientific discourse. This is perhaps partially due to the personalities and interests of the authors of these texts, but it also shows a practice in transition, as medical language and objective accounts begin to outnumber the personal and emotional accounts.

An example of a rather literary author is Charles D. Meigs, a Philadelphia physician who published several texts from the 1830s to the 1850s. Meigs' work was popular during his lifetime, but has been criticized as "marred by vanity and verbosity" by the early twentieth century's most popular textbook author, J. Whitridge Williams (qtd. in Speert 128). The profession had changed enough in fifty years that Meigs' style was considered outdated by William's scientific standards.

Meigs' case histories are characterized by personal accounts, a narrative quality, and the same attention to personal reactions that we saw in Bard's early cases. Meigs does not hesitate to include his reactions to the cases he attends, nor does he exclude what seems to be unnecessary information about the patient. The following excerpt describes his reaction to a patient's suffering:

> I think one of the most fearful instances of human agony that my eyes have ever witnessed, was that of a lady in North Sixth Street, Mrs. Th. S—y, who, being in labor of her first child, . . . began suddenly to scream, with the greatest violence, often uttering the words. "Oh, the cramp! the cramp! the cramp!" She was indescribably agitated, her

> countenance assumed the wildest expression, ... I had, for many years, been accustomed to the cries of puerperal women, to which I had become habitually indifferent, but this case deserved to be called terrible. (48)

Clearly, Meigs had a strong reaction to his patient's suffering. In his depiction of the birth, he makes no attempt to separate his personal reactions from his scientific account. His description is highly subjective: "agony," "indescribably agitated," "wildest expression," and "terrible" are all interpretations of his patient's pain.

Meigs also includes information about his personal handling of the case that may have been better left out. He tells us that because he had not brought his forceps with him he had to wait for the husband to bring them before he could relieve the woman's suffering. For her next confinement, the woman begged him to bring his forceps, fearing she would suffer from the cramp again. He refused and it was necessary to awaken a servant and send him on the fastest horse in the house to travel the five miles to retrieve them. One has to wonder why Meigs would tell his reader about his seemingly callous refusal to bring his forceps with him. He does not explain this.

If this case is full of information about Meigs, the following has a narrative quality that belies its placement in a medical text. The case is not his, but one told him by a colleague, Dr. James. Meigs retells it with relish, and the drama, coupled with the obvious didactic purpose, must have had a great effect on his reader:

> While the persons at breakfast were conversing cheerfully, and exchanging felicitations upon the fortunate issue of affairs in the lying-in room, the nurse was heard screaming from the top of the stairs, "Doctor, doctor, for God's sake come up!" He hastened to the apartment, and the lady was lying across the bed quite dead. It was found that, soon after the doctor went below, the lady said to the nurse, "I want to get up." "But you must not get up, madam; the doctor gave a very strict charge against it," replied the nurse. "I do not care what the doctor says," rejoined the patient; and thereupon arose, and throwing her feet out of the bed, she sat on the side a few moments, reeled, and fell back in a fatal fainting fit. (346)

In the complete account of this case, we are given several of the elements of a fictional narrative. The scene is described: the doctor is enjoying breakfast downstairs while mother and child recuperate upstairs. The new mother is characterized as stubborn and willful through her "actual" recorded speech, and her subsequent disobedience. The nurse, a minor character, though significant to the doctor's interpretation, is at the least ineffectual. The doctor is depicted as knowledgeable, correct, and totally blameless in the woman's death. The plot is fairly complex: the doctor has successfully delivered a healthy baby, issued orders to both the new mother and the nurse about getting up, and retired to the dining room to share breakfast with the family. The disobedient patient refuses to listen to his orders, and by getting up causes her death.

Once the story has been told, the reader is treated to Meigs' interpretation of the incident in the form of a "medical" conclusion that reads more like a moral than science:

> The remarks of Dr. James, as he related the occurrence to me, made upon my mind a deep impression of the vast consequence of careful and well-timed instruction of the nurses; who, if they could have the dangers of mismanagement fully exposed to them, would surely avoid some accidents that every now and then are attended with shocking results. (Meigs 346)

Other case histories cited in Meigs do show the adoption of scientific discourse. In the following excerpt, we can see the doctor using scientific terminology to objectify the subject of his investigation. She is presented as a case of what Meigs calls "procrastination of the term" and though the doctor comments on her pain, unlike Meigs, he doesn't appear to be affected by it. In contrast to Meigs' characterization of his patient's suffering as "agony" in the earlier case history, this doctor's use of the term "acute" reflects an attempt to achieve a scientific description of the woman's condition:

> She was laboring under a decided hectical fever [wasting or consumptive] and irritation, that had already very much reduced her flesh and strength. She obtained but little sleep, and had a poor appetite. She daily suffered acute pains in the abdomen. . . . The os uteri was found to be not dilated, though the cervix was fully

> developed, having lost entirely its tubular or cylindrical form. The form of the abdominal tumor was *conical*, the umbilicus being at the apex of the cone. . . .
>
> She remained in the ward, suffering daily and nightly with abdominal pains, until she fell into labor. . . . I sat up with her all night, being deeply interested to observe all the phenomena of the case. (233)

Though this case history shows the emergence of the objectification that scientific terms made possible, the subjective influence remains. The account is of a supposed fourteen-month pregnancy, but after listing all of the symptoms the woman displayed during labor and delivery, the doctor does not interpret this evidence, or use it to explain the length of the term. Had his account achieved complete objectivity, he would have relied upon the medical evidence to prove or disprove the purported length of the pregnancy. Instead, he adds a disclaimer at the end of the history attesting to the fact that he is relying solely on the patient's statement about when she became pregnant. He offers the following as support to her testimony: "She had the appearance of perfect candor and sincerity in all that she said about it. . . " (234). Rather than relying on the scientific evidence, he gives the reader a highly subjective judgment of the woman's veracity. We are never told why the rest of the medical information is given, or of its connection to the length of her pregnancy.

In his attitudes about science and propriety, Meigs was very representative of his profession at the time. In the introduction to *Obstetrics: The Science and Art*, first published in 1849, Meigs expresses the same value placed on the scientific approach to obstetrics as seen in earlier works, and the same concern for the propriety of male-midwifery:

> It is the Science of the practitioner that raises him immeasurably above the most dextrous midwives of the land, dexterity which indeed does not prevent their ignorance from rendering them unsafe depositories of such important interests as those that concern the conservation of our wives and daughters, and their little children. An accoucheur who is merely dextrous, and who is not acquainted with the scientific parts of his profession, may be in a manner superior to the midwife, but in some regards he is inferior; since to his

> employment, his sex is an objection, which ought to be waived only in consideration of his Scholarship. (viii)

It is obvious where Meigs' loyalties lie; he is definitely aligned on the side of science. His views on morality, however, make him uncomfortable with the untrained male midwife. His views on propriety also do not allow him to approve of the use of living women to aid the instruction of medical students. To do so would be to violate the female modesty and chastity that are the "very corner-stone of civilization and order. . ." (qtd. in Speert 78). Thus, in the middle of the century, attitudes about female modesty persisted, and doctors still had to strike a careful balance in their work in order to avoid public criticism.

In relating a case about injury to the female genitalia, Meigs clearly illustrates this dilemma. First, in regards to some plates he has included and discussed, he says:

> The question might be asked, why I should have placed these illustrations in my book, since such drawings, to say the least, seem fit to make the cheek tingle with shame. I am quite conscious that a book of medical practice ought to be written with a decent regard to decency. . . . (104)

Meigs rationalizes his choices by invoking the need to instruct the student properly. His desire to teach wins out and he recounts the following case:

> Mrs. –, the mother of four children, returned to her home from a ride on horseback. The servant brought a common country chair for her to dismount. The chair terminated in two sharp turned tops. When the lady was ready, she threw herself from the saddle, and as her food lighted on the edge of the chair, carelessly held by the groom, it turned forwards, and she fell. The sharp turned top of the chair was driven against her riding skirt, and forced her clothing just against the under edge of the arch of the pubis. In a moment she was streaming with blood, and being taken to her apartment, she bled until she fainted. . . . (104)

After citing another, similar case, in which a woman is injured after her "night vase" breaks under her weight, Meigs is compelled to stop his explanation of the potential causes of such injuries. Some are simply too embarrassing and improper to relate, even in a medical book. He apologizes once more:

> I shall not detain the Student to speak of other causes that might give rise to severe bleeding, in these tissues, it is enough to have called his attention to the general facts in which he will find not only the indications of his practice, but my apology for introducing in this work a topic so unacceptable. (105)

Attitudes about "unmentionable" topics and practices that are similar to Meigs' can be seen in the reaction of the medical community in Buffalo when, in January, 1850, Dr. John Platt White allowed twenty members of his graduating class to examine a young woman about to give birth (Speert 78). The woman was unmarried, and presumably White chose her because it was less of an assault on propriety for his students to examine a woman whose morals were already in question. He also provided her with a place to stay until she delivered, free medical care, and a ten dollar honorarium (78). These provisions probably enticed her to agree, whereas a married woman would have no need of the shelter or the honorarium, and would be sure to refuse to be examined for fear that the community would ostracize her.

The reaction to White's demonstration was swift and hostile. Seventeen of Buffalo's forty physicians signed a letter published in the *Buffalo Medical Journal* that said of the demonstration: "[W]e deem it unnecessary for the purpose of teaching, unprofessional in manner, and grossly offensive alike to morality and common decency" (qtd. in Speert 79). Another protest printed in the *Louisville Medical Journal* stated that "we do not like to see this excessive flirtation with modesty, introduced into medical teaching" (qtd. in Speert 79). The matter was referred to the AMA, which declared that a competent physician should be prepared to deliver from touch alone, having learned all he needed from textbook discussions, medical plates and mannequins (Speert 79). Though it created this fierce outcry, White's demonstration also broke the last taboo, and by the end of the century, clinical experience had become an integral part of obstetrical training.

The acceptance of clinical experience could not have been achieved without the influence of the case history. When doctors like Meigs overcame their scruples and wrote about "unmentionable" cases, they taught their students that such discussions were necessary to the profession. Such discussions went from being tolerated to accepted to expected. The students would look upon the next step, examining live patients, as an expected evolution in their training, taking them beyond the text of the case history and into the real world of its application.

Before doctors could examine women on a routine basis, the women had to be willing to submit to such examinations. Here the case history was also instrumental because it helped to change women's attitudes about medical treatment. The reproduction of case histories in women's handbooks facilitated this change in attitude. The title page of C. Morrill, M.D.'s 1856 *Physiology of Woman and Her Diseases* states that the topic has been "adapted to the instruction of females, and professional reading." In the dedication to the book entitled "False Delicacy and Notions on Anatomy and Physiology" the author has taken care to defend his discussion of such a delicate topic. In this paragraph, the author states that those who believe it is improper to show plates of the female anatomy to the youth of America are wrong. He believes that "[t]he more we attempt to conceal from children or others, the greater is their curiosity, and the stronger their desire to gratify it unobserved. Such is the law of perverted nature." Morrill bemoans the fact that "[a] medical man is rarely consulted till the health is gone; . . ." (11). His solution is to educate women, not so they can treat themselves, but so that they will call upon scientifically trained doctors and follow their advice when consulted.

Before he could convince women of this need, however, Morrill had to convince them that the book itself was an acceptable instrument of knowledge. After explaining that the primary end of a woman's existence is to propagate the species, and that her good influence over her family rests upon her charms, themselves dependent on good health, Morrill asks how a woman will know how to discharge this important duty without proper education. He asks his reader whether "he whose heart and head are better adapted to his high and responsible calling, from an absurd subjection to blind conventionalism, [will] oppose a sincere and honest effort for her instruction?" (10). Once he calls upon those "better adapted" to make such decisions (medical colleagues, husbands and fathers?), he concludes:

> It must be conceded, then, that woman ought to be educated in the physiology and nature of her organization, and the diseases to which

> she is incident. Her own welfare requires this; and not her own merely but the good of her offspring; and in fine, the proper development of the physical and moral powers of our whole race depends upon the conduct of the female before marriage, during pregnancy, suckling, and afterwards. (11)

By making the moral development of the human race dependent on the proper education of women, Morrill managed to stand the propriety argument on its head. Anyone concerned with true morality would see that the only way to accomplish it was to put "within her [woman's] reach those truths concerning her organization which have been elicited by the patient investigations of the accomplished medical men, who have in every age of the world devoted their lives to these subjects . . . " (11).

Morrill's argument was the same advanced by the health reform movement of the nineteenth century. Reformers argued that only through knowledge about physiology would women be equipped to care for their own and their family's health. By using the commonly held belief that women were moral superiors to men, the reformers added health to women's sphere of influence (Morantz "Making Women Modern" 351). The arguments to the contrary depicted women as highly susceptible to suggestion and weak-minded; reading highly sensational novels, for example could lead a women to idolize her passions and succumb to the first opportunisitic scoundrel who came along (Kerber 244). Potential readers of Morrill's handbook—mothers and fathers contemplating giving it to their daughters to read—would want to be sure that it would not excite prurient interests and, by doing so, ruin its reader's virtue. To assure his audience that the author has not left propriety completely behind, Morrill explains that he has "also labored, as far as consistent with truthful exposition, to avoid shocking the prejudices or delicacy of the reader" (12).

Perhaps because his handbook will be more controversial than a medical text by virtue of its expanded audience, Morrill must always balance his concern for delicacy with his mission to educate women in "proper management." Proper management tips the scales when he explains that he must discuss one topic that has been ignored by others: masturbation. Rather than apologizing for his embarrassing subject matter as Meigs does, Morrill tells his reader that "[w]e should consider ourselves highly culpable, notwithstanding we may shock the prejudices of the reader, did we neglect, in this place, to point out a most prominent cause of precocious puberty in young females" (63). He explains that, while other authors have ignored the subject, he cannot, since he sees the health of thousands of youth "sacrificed to its shrine" (63). Later in the text, to reinforce his condemnation of this practice, he cites the case history of a young girl whose nymphomania he attributes to enlarged genital organs, a condition he speculates may have been caused by her practice of what he has earlier referred to as "artificial indulgence" (63):

> The genital organs of some women, acquire such a preponderance, as to make it always impossible for them to control the intensity of the erotic flame which devours them; such was the young girl of whom Buffon speaks: "I have seen, and I have regarded her as a singular phenomenon, a girl of twelve years of age, a dark brunette, of a bright and highly colored complexion, of small stature, but already fully formed, with a rounded neck and embonpoint [a euphemism for plumpness, perhaps referring to her breasts], perform the most indecent action at the simple appearance of a man; nothing could control her in this, neither the presence of her mother, nor remonstrances, nor punishments. Yet she did not lose her reason, and the attack, which was carried to such a point as to be frightful, ceased the moment that she remained alone with women." (177-178)

Morrill's treatment for the enlarged clitoris is "cooling and astringent applications with saline purging. . . at the same time avoiding exciting food, indolence, improper associations, sentimental reading, etc." (276). When these treatments fail:

> amputation of the salient organ should always be recommended, which is performed without subsequent inconvenience to the female, and with producing very little pain. Thus, it is consoling to reflect, that the female may be rid of a disgusting depravity, with perfect safety. Instances are not wanting, in which, girls have been entirely cured of masturbation by this operation, which had resisted all other means. In such cases a competent surgeon should always be consulted. (276)

Most of Morrill's case histories are selected for a similar didactic function. The following case teaches women to avoid the bad judgment demonstrated by the mother in the story, and not incidentally, to be sure to choose a scientifically trained doctor:

> Dr. Dewees mentions the . . . sad fate of a "most amiable and interesting young creature," for whom he was requested to prescribe for the expected menses. She was in perfect health, and had not a mark of womanhood—though she was fifteen years of age—and this was all that could be urged by the mother in favor of an attempt to "bring down her courses." (Morrill 96)

The doctor explains to the mother that there is nothing medical to be done in the situation, but six months later he finds the daughter ill and then dead as a result of the oil of savin (the dried tops of the juniper shrub, highly poisonous and often used to induce abortion) supplied by a quack:

> It seems that the mother, with the view of producing the menstrual discharge, had procured some medicine of a quack, which, upon giving according to his directions, produced fever, loss of appetite, and vomiting; she again called upon the "Doctor," and he encouraged her to persevere with the medicine, saying that the fever, etc., was an effort of nature for the end proposed—"she persevered, fatally persevered; for in a few days more she lost her lovely and only daughter." (Morrill 96)

The message to the female reader is that it is important to listen to the scientifically trained doctor's advice. Consulting with a quack can be deadly. The author makes a connection between practicing for the sole purpose of acquiring wealth and "deficient qualifications" (Morrill 96). Thus, a well-trained doctor will also be one for whom the patient's best interests come first and will therefore be the only trustworthy choice.

As in Meigs, in this case the patient and her mother are given characterizations; the daughter is a most amiable and interesting creature, while the mother is willful and negligent in her single-minded desire to induce her daughter's menses. The doctor creates a very sympathetic ethos for himself by so representing the dead girl, and by expressing his fatherly concern over this type of unscientific practice.

This focus allows him to retain an emphasis on the didactic purpose of warning women away from "quack" practitioners. What he does not discuss in this case is the possibility that the girl was pregnant and the oil of savin was used to induce an early abortion—a method of birth control quite common in the nineteenth century.

Morrill does, however, address abortion, and his discussion is representative of his profession's growing hostility toward this method of birth control. Until the early 1800s, abortion had been a common form of birth control in the American colonies, which had followed British common law allowing abortions until the advent of quickening (Mohr 16). Only by detecting movement could a pregnancy be validated, and this method certainly put the woman in control of her pregnancy since only she could know when the child began to move. Early arguments and laws against abortion were actually in response to the use of poisonous concoctions like the oil of savin discussed above. The first law passed against abortion simply set penalties for using poisons after quickening (21). The movement against abortion changed when it also became part of a strategy to eliminate practitioners who were not scientifically trained—especially the midwife (37). Because these alternative practitioners were likely to be providing the means for abortion, outlawing it became a way to outlaw them.

Morrill's views on abortion also reflect the growing moral outrage that doctors were beginning to feel for the practice. Perhaps because they had a better understanding of the genesis of life, they were increasingly uncomfortable with ending it prematurely (35-36). Another possible motive for objection was adherence to eugenicist views that the "wrong" (lower-class, immigrants, and the unhealthy) people were reproducing and the "right" (middle- and upper-class) were not. The fear of "race suicide" was prevalent in the nineteenth century and doctors counseled against birth control for their privileged patients who had already shown what seemed to be an alarming drop in the birth rate. (Gordon "Why Nineteenth-Century Feminists" 43). For whichever of these reasons, Morrill had great antipathy for abortionists or for those who enlisted their services. In his introduction, he characterizes abortionists as "female fiends" (10) and later as ". . . degraded wretches, not less criminal than the unnatural women, who are not ashamed to submit to their disgusting ministrations, . . . " (316). The result of these attempts to abort is that, in most cases, the woman is not only unsuccessful at ending the pregnancy, but if she lives, she suffers terrible physical consequences.

> I once prescribed for a female, in whom such attempts had brought on a flooding which conducted her to the verge of the grave; she suffered horribly from pain in the interior of the pelvis for two months, notwithstanding which abortion did not take place, and she is now a prey to a large ulcer of the neck of the womb. I opened the body of an unhappy creature who suffered from like attempts, which did not succeed any better than the one above mentioned. (316)

In another set of cases, Morrill warns his audience against the quack practitioner who attempts to cure cancer with caustic substances. "For the purpose of guarding our readers against a certain class of empirics who infest the country, professing to cure cancer, we quote the following sensible and very true remarks of Dr. Dixon's, upon the subject of 'cancer plasters'" (256). Morrill cites Dixon at length about the pain and suffering that will be caused by these false remedies, bolstering his argument that the surgeon's knife is a far better option:

> It is but a short time since the coroner was called to inspect the body of the unfortunate mother of a family in this city, who had been poisoned by the absorption of arsenic from a plaster applied by one of these wretched traffickers in human life. We were called to see another, who had lost an eyelid by the corrosive action of a similar preparation; and this too, as she assured us, for a trifling enlargement of a little blood-vessel—'a mere speck, the size of a pin's head,' as she expressed it—that had remained from infancy to her twenty-fifth year! What more conclusive evidence that it was not a cancer, could there be? Cancer never attacks an infant, as everyone knows. (256-7)

The case histories presented in Morrill are mostly devoid of the early scientific language found in some of the cases included by Bard and Meigs. Morrill, however, has a different audience and purpose. Because he wants to convince women to see medically trained doctors, and to act in a moral fashion, his purpose is more didactic than informative, despite his statements in the introduction. It serves his purpose to fill the case histories with the horrible results of the improper actions of both women and quacks. The language is highly charged and seems calculated to create fear. Normal woman, "the most beautiful object of creation," with her "attractive charms which act as an undying stimulus to man," (7) is contrasted with the "disgusting ministrations" (316) of the "female fiends" (10) who perform abortions. The woman who dies at the hands of a quack is an "unfortunate mother," (265) while she who dies after procuring an abortion is an "unhappy creature" (316).

Morrill also plays with language, in some cases to make the problem appear worse, and in some perhaps to avoid his own questionable interest in the topic. Masturbation sounds much worse when it is called "the degrading vice of artificial indulgence," (63). The term "embonpoint," (177) used to tone down his description of the young nymphomaniac's breasts, allows him to talk about her lasciviousness without sounding guilty of the same crime himself. In this same case we are simply told the young girl performed an indecent action, but we are never told what it is. Perhaps by allowing the reader to fill in this blank herself, Morrill accomplished his purpose of warning women away from any type of "inflamed" thought, while avoiding going into the "dangerous" details himself.

If Morrill flirts with the titillating nature of the material he includes in his book, a later author, Seth Pancoast, M.D., seems to revel in it. His book, *The Ladies' New Medical Guide*, published in Philadelphia in 1890, is a ladies' handbook intended for "every female interested in the health, beauty, longevity, happiness, and general well-being of her sex" (Pancoast vii). The publisher's preface informs us that Dr. Pancoast has written the book after "having his mind early drawn to the physical perfection and beauty of women, . . ." (v). The text itself, however, does not focus on the questions the typical woman would probably have asked about pregnancy and childbirth. Instead, Pancoast seems much more interested in the bizarre and freakish.

Embedded in the first section, which deals with woman's anatomy, are chapters on hermaphrodism, the moral institution of marriage, and woman's proper sphere of action. Though hardly medical, the chapters on marriage and woman's sphere of action are understandable in a nineteenth-century handbook that also has a moral purpose. The chapter on hermaphrodism indicates a keen interest in distinctions between genders, and the freakish, side-show attractions that doctors before him had studied in order to determine what truly separates the masculine and feminine genders. In fact, a closer look at the case studies Pancoast includes suggests that he is using the guise of "glorious science" to discuss topics that seem both inappropriate for a woman's handbook and, that are perhaps indicative of his own prurient interests.

Of the 112 cases included in the book, 26 are about emotional shocks to the mother causing bizarre birth defects. Twenty are about hermaphrodites; seventeen are about monstrous births like Siamese twins; twelve are about mothers killing their children by nursing them while upset; and nine are about superfoetation (in which the author proves that a woman can be impregnated more than once during a pregnancy). The remaining 28 cases also illustrate very unusual situations such as very old men fathering children, women purported to have given birth to as many as 365 children (at once!), and early puberty (ten months old). None of these cases would have been of particular interest to the normal woman looking for information about how best to manage her pregnancy and most of them would have made her more frightened than if she had no information at all.

For example, the readers of this book could learn that "a woman who had longed for a lobster brought forth a child resembling one of these animals" (206) and "another woman had a female child, the head of which looked like a shell-fish, (a bi-valve that opens and shuts its mouth), which was caused by the mother having a strong desire for mussels during pregnancy" (206-7). For the reader not frightened by fish stories, there's one about the woman who, upon seeing a criminal broken on the wheel, gave birth to an idiot child with similar broken bones (205). Finally, one of the most morbid tells of a pregnant woman who longed to bite the shoulder of a baker she knew:

> The husband wishing to gratify this morbid fancy of his wife, hired the man to submit to the operation. The woman made two bites, and so severe, that he would not allow her to try again. She gave birth to three children—one dead and two living. In this case it seemed to require a bite for each child to remove the morbid disease of the mind. Two bites being granted and the third refused, the refusal no doubt caused the third child to fall victim to the morbid mind of the mother. (207)

Once the reader had learned that she had to worry about what she craved and what she saw during pregnancy, she could be further frightened by Pancoast's discussion of nursing, in which he warns mothers not to nurse their children while they are upset about anything. The cases he includes are graphic examples of the medical view of women as flawed both physically and emotionally. In the following case, a woman "kills" her child by nursing while in an agitated state:

> While in [a] state of strong excitement, the mother took up her child from the cradle, where it lay playing and in the most perfect health, never having had a moment's illness. She gave it the breast, and in so doing sealed its fate. In a few minutes the infant left off suckling, became restless, panted and sank dead upon its mother's bosom. (299)

Of all of the odd cases included in the book, the ones about hermaphrodism are perhaps the most inappropriate to a woman's handbook. They are also the most bizarre and perhaps even titillating for both author and reader alike. Pancoast discusses both spurious and true hermaphrodism and sample cases for both follow:

> Otto has reported a remarkable case of a person who had lived for ten long years in a state of wedlock with three different men. At the age of thirty-five her third husband brought an action of divorce against her, alleging that she was afflicted with some sexual infirmity, which rendered the connubial act on his part extremely difficult and painful. On examination being made by two physicians, they decided that she was not a female but a male. The members of the Royal Medical College of Silesia subsequently confirmed this decision. The penis was imperforated and about two inches in length. There was a perineal fissure forming a false vagina, that was sufficient to receive the penis of the husband for an inch and a half in depth. The general conformation of this individual was strong and muscular, although the beard was thin and soft. The face, mammae, chest, pelvis and extremities were masculine. (142-143)

Imagine the images that would be formed in the reader's mind upon reading this story. How would the nineteenth-century woman have responded to this discussion? Surely it would have offended her modesty, regardless of how open-minded she was toward obtaining medical information about pregnancy. In virtually every case about hermaphrodites, the length of the penis/clitoris is discussed, the individual's sexual proclivities mentioned, and most of the other organs and their functions described in depth. A case of "true" hermaphrodism is a good example of these features:

> An interesting case of Hermaphrodism has been given by Dr. Hendry of New York, in a letter dated from Lisbon in 1807. The subject was Portuguese, aged twenty-eight years, of a tall and slender muscular figure. The penis and testicles were in their usual situation, and in form and size resembled those of a male about the same age. The urethra extended to about one-third the length of the penis. The beard had a tendency to grow, but was kept cut short. The female parts resembled those of a well-formed person, except the labia, which were not prominent. The external organs appeared to be situated near the rectum. The breasts were small, voice and manners like those of a female. She menstruated regularly; was twice pregnant, and miscarried in the third and fourth month of gestation. During copulation, the penis became erect, but there never was a desire for copulation with the female sex. (148)

Pancoast's book of bizarre cases shows how far the discussion of gynecology had progressed from Bard's distinctly personal account of his reaction to a retroverted uterus, Meigs' blushing apologies, White's controversial student demonstration, and Morrill's impassioned defense of educating women in physiology. Though atypical, Pancoast demonstrates that this type of discussion had become far more accepted by both the medical establishment and the general public, which would have formed the readership for his woman's handbook.

Male-authored medical texts and handbooks were by no means the only material on women's health and reproduction published and/or distributed in the nineteenth century. The health reform movement stimulated a great deal of writing on physiology, health, sex, and reproductive control. By the middle of the nineteenth century "books, pamphlets, tracts, and booklets ranging from a dozen pages to several hundred, some solely text and others with dozens of engravings or elaborate colored and fold-out illustrations, circulated" (Brodie 202). The authors of these texts were varied, ranging from English feminist Annie Besant's neo-Malthusian[3] *The Law of Population* to Lydia Pinkham's advertisements for her vegetable compound (180, 190). Much of this literature has been lost, however, and texts that appear to have been written by women may have in fact been written by men using female pen names to boost credibility with their audiences (184).

A text that appears to have been popular at the end of the nineteenth century is Dr. Alice B. Stockham's *Tokology: A Book for Every Woman*, published in 1884. Women surveyed at the end of the century listed the text as one they had read for knowledge of sexual physiology (Brodie 202). Stockham's text is strictly practical, with sections on proper dress and shoes, exercise, and diet. She includes whole chapters on constipation, proper ventilation, indigestion and nausea, and the various other symptoms of pregnancy. The last chapter provides recipes for her fruit and rice diet.

The case histories included in this volume are also quite different from those in Pancoast's handbook and the medical texts we have examined. Stockham uses cases to illustrate the points she makes about dress, exercise and diet, and in each we hear the woman's voice speaking, not the doctor's. All are personal accounts told to the doctor, or sent in the form of a letter. None is quoted from another medical authority. A good example is a letter sent by a Mrs. C., published verbatim in the book:

> "This is to verify that I know what Dr. Stockham teaches in regard to "Fruit Diet" is true. When pregnant with my last child, accidentally I lived upon rice and fruit, and my child was born comparatively without pain or sensible effort; could not get a physician in time, nor did I need one. In four previous deliveries I had physicians with me over twenty-four hours, and had prolonged and severe labors. I can account for the difference only in the fruit and rice diet." (122)

Stockham's book is definitely a woman's book for women. Her aim is to educate women so that they can better care for themselves; her discussion of specific gynecological matters is limited to practical issues. This same pattern is followed in other women's handbooks authored by women. Mrs. Prudence Saur's *Maternity: A Book for Every Wife and Mother*, published in 1896, also illustrates the homeopathic approach to medicine. Dr. Saur takes great care to print her qualifications on the title page of the book, but she does not try to establish herself as a scientist by using case histories to prove her points. Instead we find only three actual case histories cited and these are used to explain the effect of maternal influence on the fetus, and the positive results of a fruit diet very similar to Stockham's. A chapter titled "The Relation of Health to Beauty," contributed by Dr. Ruth Blake to *The New Tokology: Mother and Child Culture*, published in 1902, addresses the dangers of the corset. "A woman who laces tightly cannot bear a healthy child, and her foolish belief that such a distorted figure as she manages to produce is beautiful, leads to much suffering" (407). Finally, another turn of the century publication, *Perfect Womanhood for Maidens-Wives-Mothers* (1903) by Mary Melendy, M.D., Ph. D., is a virtual reprint of Saur's book (without acknowledgment), citing the same three cases and no more.

By the end of the nineteenth century, the most significant change in the birth process had already occurred. Birth had been redefined as a disease, and control over its management placed firmly in the hands of medical science. This pathological view of birth sets the stage for the medical intervention that characterizes birth management in the twentieth century. Without the change in attitude toward the medical profession's involvement in birth, and toward birth itself, the reproductive technologies that are becoming commonplace in this century could never have been conceived of by the women who participate in them. Chapter three demonstrates how the case history becomes a regular offering in the popular media, as it continues to create an atmosphere of acceptance for medical intervention in the creation of life.

NOTES

1. Male practitioners preferred the term obstetrics because it was scientific sounding and it eliminated the gender orientation suggested by the term midwife.

2. Scientific practitioners made a distinction between women who lived a more natural and rigorous lifestyle and the more "civilized" middle- and upper-class women they attended. The gynecology textbooks of the nineteenth century often relate stories of peasant women giving birth in fields and calmly going on with their work. In contrast, refined women were seen as nervous, sickly, weak, and full of fear about childbirth.

3. Malthusians believed that the world's population would overtake the food supply and promoted reproductive control as a solution. Reproductive control was also seen as a way to improve society by limiting the reproductive

capabilities of the sick, mentally deficient and for some, the lower classes (Brodie 90-91).

CHAPTER THREE

Gynecology at the Check-out Stand

With the birth of Louise Joy Brown in 1978, the modern gynecological case history became standard fare in the lifestyles-type publication. With 179 or 20% of all articles published on reproductive technology since 1977, the lifestyles magazine has printed more on the topic than any other category. Though the lifestyles genre includes a range of personal interest publications, I have chosen to narrow the focus to the women's magazine because its audience is the prime target group for the reproductive technologies that the modern case history now promotes.

The women's magazine is an extremely appropriate place to investigate messages being sent to women about the new technologies because of the role this periodical institution has played in shaping women's views of themselves and their roles as wives and mothers. The women's magazine has worked closely with the advertising industry to promote products designed to make the American housewife the best possible wife and mother. Edward Bok, editor of *The Ladies' Home Journal* from 1889 to 1920, explained this symbiotic relationship in 1898:

> It is the growth of advertising in this country which, more than any other single element, has brought the American magazine to its present enviable position in points of literary, illustrative, and mechanical excellence. The American advertiser has made the superior American magazine of today possible. (qtd. in Wood 112)

In his history of American magazines, James Wood explains the flip-side of this relationship: "Women's magazines are likewise a valuable advertising medium. Editorial and advertising pages naturally complement each other. Love is the subject of a romantic short story; the accessories of love are for sale in the advertising pages" (127). Based on this lucrative association, one could add that the American magazine has made the superiority of the advertising business possible as well.

The case history has adapted quite well to the women's magazine, an excellent venue for selling both ideal womanhood and technology. Already a persuasive text, the case history can now draw on the women's magazines' well-established promotion of motherhood to present medical technologies as the answer to the childless woman's dreams. The change in agent from doctor to patient or her narrator makes the case history even more effective because personal accounts are both sentimental and sensational, and because the authors have a close affinity with their audience. These are women talking to women: sisters, daughters, mothers, and grandmothers sharing their stories of love, longing and courage. The stories being shared are strikingly similar in their emotional extremes, overblown language, and ubiquitous happy endings. They read like modern fairy tales, with all of the attendant elements: a woman so committed to motherhood that she endures a painful and heroic struggle to complete herself through childbirth and/or motherhood; a doctor who wields technology like a magic wand to make the childless woman's dreams come true; and the final achievement, the perfect "miracle" baby who is the inevitable result.

Who is the woman browsing through *The Ladies' Home Journal* or *Good Housekeeping* as she waits at the check-out stand during her weekly shopping expedition? Depending upon which magazine she selects, she may or may not be college-educated and her age will range from 25 to 55. She is married, with an annual household income of $40,000 per year (*Redbook* Research, 1994), and she works to help keep her family fed, housed, and financially secure (Margolis 219). Today's woman appears to have more options than her grandmother, but with these options come greater responsibilities. She not only works to provide consumer goods, but also considers a host of factors when making purchasing decisions in her capacity as the household's professional consumer. She must determine which products will be efficient, convenient, well-made, environmentally safe, and healthy.

To establish financial stability for her family, the woman at the check-1out stand may have delayed motherhood well into her thirties: "If she had children, the young woman of the 1980s was likely to have them later than her mother had done. During the 1970s, fertility dropped precipitously among women in their early twenties although it increased among women a decade older" (Woloch 533). As a result of delaying reproduction, many women ready to start families have found that they can not conceive. Extended use of birth control pills, untreated sexually transmitted diseases, pelvic inflammatory diseases, endometriosis, and the natural decline in fertility that comes with age are some of the factors that contribute to what appears to be an increase of infertility in women.

For this new problem, medical science now has a solution. Just as technology took over women's productive activities in the nineteenth century, medicine today provides a technology that can take over the twentieth-century woman's reproductive function. Added to the advertisements in the women's service magazine that promote consumer goods are case histories promoting the latest marvels of medical technology: the "miracle babies" being created in the nation's laboratories. Consumerism has come full circle; women can now purchase the technology that creates babies. They may even purchase the use of another woman's body to be used as the site of this technology and have their own genetically-related child delivered into their open but unlabored arms.

To understand the audience of the women's magazine better, a brief discussion of the more general cultural scene will illustrate how several key twentieth-century events have made this state of reproductive affairs possible. The change in attitude that came with the medicalization of birth in the nineteenth century helped to prepare the way for the emergence of reproductive technology. The view of the birth process as flawed predisposed the contemporary woman to accept infertility as a problem that must be cured by any means possible.

The birth control movement that began in the nineteenth century continued to gather strength in the twentieth for a variety of reasons. The criminalization of abortion made access to birth control even more important. The movement itself was characterized by mixed motives. Support for legalized birth control came from disparate groups. Feminists and socialists saw it as a means to free women to choose the course of their lives, while eugenicists supported it for very different reasons. They saw it as a way to limit reproduction by those they deemed unfit: the poor, and the mentally and physically defective (Woloch 365). For middle-class whites, however, many eugenicists opposed birth control because they feared it would be a means of committing "race suicide" (365). Other opponents included doctors who worried that it would demean the marriage contract and somehow violate the "sanctity of motherhood" (365). Many middle-class women also opposed legalizing birth control because they believed easy access to it would encourage promiscuity among their men (365). Crusaders against obscenity influenced the movement significantly by passing laws that prohibited the distribution of information about birth control. In 1873, Anthony Comstock, the head of the New York Society for the Suppression of Vice, persuaded Congress to outlaw the circulation of obscene literature. The passage of this law marked a turning point in anti-contraceptive legislation (Mohr 197). Comstock became a special agent for the government and zealously caught and prosecuted those who violated the new federal offense. It was now a crime to

> Sell, or offer to sell, or . . . give away, or offer to give away, or . . . have in possession with intent to sell or give away, an obscene or indecent book, pamphlet, paper, advertisement, drawing, lithograph, engraving, wood-cut, daguerrotype, photograph, stereoscopic picture, model, cast, instrument, or other article of indecent or immoral nature, or any article or medicine . . . for causing abortion. (qtd. in Mohr 196)

The law also prohibited writing, printing, or causing such items to be printed. The result of Comstock's campaign was that birth control information was not readily available to women who did not have regular family doctors to attend to their health. Lower class birth rates and maternal illness rose, while middle-class birth rates declined steadily through the 1930s, and only began to increase again with the baby boom after the second World War (Evans 238). For the middle-class woman, birth control was a means of maintaining financial stability and retaining middle-class status by limiting children to an affordable number. Thus, motherhood was promoted for the middle-class woman; using birth control simply meant she could do a better job of mothering.

For the lower-class woman, however, birth control had an entirely different meaning. Without access to birth control information or safe abortions (Margolis 42), and with no funds for regular visits to a family doctor, the large, poverty-stricken immigrant population of the country had no means by which to limit birth. For the lower-class woman, birth control meant survivial, both economic and physical (Evans 200). Many of those who promoted birth control for her, however, saw it as a way of preventing her from ever becoming a mother and thereby ensuring the quality of the race.

In 1912, Margaret Sanger, working as a public health nurse in New York's Lower East Side, witnessed the results of legal prohibitions of birth control as she nursed women back to health from botched, illegal abortions (Woloch 363). After nursing a patient named Sadie Sachs through two abortions, the last one fatal, Sanger began her lifelong crusade for contraception.[1] Success for the birth control movement was marked by a federal court decision in 1936 which made it legal for doctors to distribute birth control devices and information (443). In 1960, the birth control pill was approved by the FDA (Evans 265). Finally, Roe v. Wade legalized abortion in 1973 (Woloch 524).

These legal developments made it easier for women to have sex without bearing children. For the middle-class woman this freedom meant the opportunity to attain a higher education and, with it, a better position in the work force. At the end of World War II, however, the American housewife was asked to vacate the marketplace so that the returning troops could find employment (Woloch 472). To encourage her to go "back to the kitchen," motherhood was promoted even more assiduously than before (473). The baby boom period of the fifties and sixties is a testament to the efficacy of this movement.

Whether she was educated or not, and whether she continued to work or not, the typical woman of the fifties was still intent upon marriage and family. Her education would simply make her a more interesting wife and a better mother (500-501). Working would allow her to contribute to the family income before childbirth and after her children were reared (500). The women's magazine was a major proponent of the new domesticity, touting motherhood as a woman's only real vocation. "'Whether they work at outside jobs or not, today's young mothers find their greatest satisfaction in home, husband, and family'" (*Ladies' Home Journal* qtd. in Margolis 222).

At the same time that many women were responding to the call back to the kitchen in the forties and fifties, contemporary feminists' were critiquing the traditional family and finding it oppressive to women (Gordon "Why Nineteenth-Century Feminists" 51). Advocating a new individualism and a rejection of gender roles, many women who followed this philosophy rejected the stereotypical nurturing role reserved for women. Meanwhile, medical science had gone far beyond its nineteenth-century focus on mastering techniques for treating dangerous and painful labors. The isolation and synthesis of the female sex hormones that led to the development of the birth control pill in the 1950s also set the stage for modern reproductive technologies like in vitro fertilization. The pill made it possible for feminists to choose not to have children, facilitating their rejection of traditional family structures. Historian Linda Gordon argues that "feminism has undermined the family as it once existed faster than it has been able to substitute more egalitarian communities." She calls for "a feminist program and philosophy that defends individual rights and also builds constructive bonds between individuals" (51). This reconstruction of family bonds has occurred to some extent with men and women who choose alternative lifestyles. While feminists tend to criticize the negative effects of reproductive technologies, there are those who support technologies that make it possible for single, lesbian, and gay people to bring children into the alternative lifestyles they have chosen.

Because reproductive technologies can help non-traditional and traditional families alike, the market for these services is booming. Middle-class women and their partners are a ready and accepting audience, with what appears to be a growing incidence of infertility, a strong desire to procreate genetically, and the well-trained consumer's desire for perfection. Single, gay, and lesbian people who wish to have families are interested in the technologies because they can now create alternative families. This demand for services, combined with technical developments in reproductive technologies and genetic research, means that gynecological practitioners are now in possession of all of the tools necessary to manipulate every stage of the production of life. Soon our scientists will have the ability to detect and eliminate the genes that cause diseases like cancer, Alzheimer's disease, muscular dystrophy, and Tay Sachs. Will we also learn to eliminate physical and psychological traits considered by some to be undesirable as well? Will the next "dis-eases" on the list be traits like eye color, gender, race, and homosexuality? (How ironic that would be for the gay and lesbian supporters of reproductive technologies.)

This manipulation of life cannot be practiced without women's acceptance and participation. In the women's magazine, the case history has been an integral tool in the promotion of the new technologies. It supports the medical goal of unravelling the mysteries of reproduction by selling the new technologies as medical miracles. With the women's magazine still hard at work promoting motherhood for the woman of the nineties, it comes as no surprise that the case history performs the dual role of selling both motherhood and technology within its pages. Case histories are presented as success stories that rarely, if ever, address the underlying ethical and moral questions they should inevitably raise. Instead, they reinforce the belief that women's lives will be unfulfilled if they do not reproduce, emphasizing this reproductive goal over any potential damage to the woman's body. Technology offers the medical help to accomplish what is still considered (at least within the pages of the women's magazine) to be the ultimate expression of true womanhood: maternity. The women in these stories are presented as heroic sufferers who would endure any amount of pain to attain their goal of motherhood. This emphasis on women's instinctive need to reproduce helps to maintain an underlying definition of women as incubators, valued solely for their ability to nurture new life. Ironically, the new technologies take reproduction out of women's bodies, and place control over it firmly in the hands of the quality-conscious field of medicine.

Representing motherhood to the reader of the women's magazine as the most vital accomplishment of her life is not a difficult task. Women's magazines have been dedicating themselves to the goal of helping their reader to become the best housewife and mother possible since the nineteenth century. The magazines are filled with stories whose morals offer advice on how to properly fulfill the duties of wife and mother.

Goodey's Lady's Book is an excellent example of a popular nineteenth-century publication that promoted ideal femininity. A women's magazine which flourished under the editorship of Sarah Josepha Hale from 1837 to 1877 (Zophy 1-2), *Goodey's* large, middle-class readership provided Hale with a forum for the editorials she used to promote her ideas on the appropriate expression of womanhood during the Victorian era (3). She believed that women should exhibit the four basic characteristics that define what is called the "cult of true womanhood": purity, piety, domesticity, and submission (Welter 103-113, Zophy 44). With a peak circulation of a half-million readers in 1869 (Zophy 50), Sarah Hale had an excellent forum in which to express her ideals. This she did by printing a combination of her own editorials, short fiction, poetry, feature articles and essays, fashion plates and engravings (49).

A fictional story that teaches how important submission is to the ideal wife was printed in the May 1844 edition of *Goodey's Magazine and Lady's Book*. Titled "I Will!" the story tells of a young girl who is worried that her fiancé will prove to be an overbearing husband. Her aunt, concerned that her niece will make the same mistake she did, decides to tell her the story of her own marriage. It seems that as a young bride, she stood up to her husband: when he forbade her to see a friend he didn't like, she refused to obey. He left the home and ten days later she received word that he was on his deathbed. Though not explicitly stated, his subsequent death is attributed by implication to her disobedience. Her advice to her niece is to "[a]void carefully, religiously avoid, setting yourself in opposition to your husband" (Arthur 215). The niece follows her aunt's advice, and she and her husband live happily ever after: "now they smoothly glide along the stream of life blessed indeed in all their marriage relations" (215).

Another fictional story, titled "Baby-Visiting," exemplifies the ideal traits of domesticity by telling the story of a sensible young mother. Mrs. Dunham sends her three children and their nurse off to several of her friends' homes on their first rounds of visits. At each household, the reader is treated to an example of bad mothering. The first friend refuses to see the children at all because she "would as soon admit so many spaniels; and as to having my carpets soiled and my bijouterie broken by other people's children, that's out of the question" (Annan 266). The second mother, Mrs. Fenwick, is obsessed with clothing her children in the most luxuriant materials she can find, and she criticizes the simple clothing Mrs. Dunham prefers. When Mrs. Fenwick's children enter the room, it is evident that they are spoiled brats, arguing and fighting amongst themselves. They then turn to the Dunham children to continue their fight (268). The nurse takes the children and leaves, but not before the Fenwicks have influenced little Lizzy Dunham, who produces a temper tantrum on the street over her plain bonnet (269). On they go, from house to house, being stuffed with sweets, quizzed by a woman who is obsessed with education, and exposed to illness by a negligent mother. When they finally return home and Mrs. Dunham learns of their adventures, she wisely decides that this will be their last visiting expedition.

Nearly one hundred years later, we find the case history still teaching submission and domesticity in the *Ladies' Home Journal* (*LHJ*) and in the context of obtaining medical care. A case history that appeared in the April 1949 edition illustrates how well accepted medical birthing practices had become by the end of the first half of the century. It also encourages women to comply with their doctor's authoritative choices about childbirth. The author, Betsy Marvin McKinney, tells the story of the birth of her third child. After two anesthetized births, the author decides to have her third child "naturally." She cites a book by Grantly Dick Read, *Childbirth Without Fear*, and chronicles her experience (116). Reed's book and his theories about drug-free childbirth were somewhat controversial. Many of his colleagues refused to work with him and thought his advocacy against drugs to be harmful to women. McKinney convinces her doctor to go along with her plan. At the hospital she is viewed as something of a medical curiosity by those who attend her. She tells her story about her "desire to witness the birth of [her] child as a rational [i.e. undrugged] woman" in order to help other women to experience the same pleasure that she did (116).

Though on the surface this account may seem to call accepted obstetrical practices into question, McKinney does not question the necessity for medical attention or for the doctor's approval of her choice to give birth without drugs. She has her child at the hospital with both an internist and her obstetrician in attendance. The story reinforces the normality of the hospital birth, and simply modifies it by showing that with doctor approval anesthesia may not always be necessary. McKinney has acted quite correctly. She has submissively asked for her doctor's permission for her unusual treatment, and she has done so to maximize her enjoyment of childbirth, the experience that most fully defines her domesticity.

Another group of case histories appears in *LHJ* in 1950 in its "Tell Me Doctor" series, authored by Henry B. Safford, M.D. He recounts the stories of several women who come to his office with gynecological complaints. While he treats them, he gives a running commentary on what he is doing and why. His explanations are often very medical i.e.

"paroxysmal vasomotor dilation of the surface vessels" for hot flashes (#10 31). This series is an interesting hybrid of the scientific approach to gynecological treatment and the human interest type of account we see in McKinney's story.

Though Safford's primary objective seems to be presenting medical information for his reader, his moral and social values are at best thinly veiled, at worst overt and obvious. His patients are linguistic constructs, easily manipulated to show his approval or disapproval of their actions. He asks the patients questions about abortions with a disapproving frown, and when one woman asks his opinion about artificial insemination, he hesitates, then responds that it is only acceptable when the husband's sperm is used. Certainly the purity ethic still holds true for Dr. Safford.

The eighth case in the series is a good example of the doctor's expectation that his patients will submit to male authority—in this case the medical authority. It begins with the caption: "I guess I had to learn the hard way, Doctor. And now that I've learned—it's too late" (Safford #8 31). In this case, a woman has come to the doctor's office with a problem she has had for two years. Though she has seen other doctors, no one has cured her and she has discontinued treatment. She appears to be rather ignorant. When the doctor asks what the previous diagnosis was, she says "'[s]omething about my tubes. I didn't understand what'" (31). When he finally gets it out of her that she has gonorrhea, he chastises her severely for discontinuing the treatments. "'You were a foolish woman not to have done as you were advised—criminally foolish! . . . You never would have gotten away with it in this town!'" (31).

The characterization of this woman as foolish is reinforced when the doctor begins to explain the nature of the infection to her and she says she doesn't understand him. He responds "'I'll take a couple of minutes to explain, even though it can't make much difference to you'" (31). The doctor explains the etiology of the disease, in medical terms, then asks "'[h]ave I made it clear what has taken place?'" (212). The patient, obviously lost in the language, answers "'I guess I'll have to believe what you tell me Doctor. They said you knew your business'" (212).

Next the doctor tells her that because of the seriousness of the disease, all of her reproductive organs will have to be removed. When the patient objects, he tells her that she will never have children, that her ovaries are gone, and her "'uterus is of no use'" (213). By the time the doctor is finished explaining her condition to her, the patient is subdued by his knowledge and compliant in the face of his authority. Finally showing the submissiveness that could have saved her reproductive organs, she tugs "silently at the corner of her handkerchief" and makes the statement that serves as the caption to this case: "'I guess I had to learn the hard way. And now that I've learned—it's too late'" (213).

In another case the doctor shows his almost god-like knowledge of the human body when his patient walks into the office and he says he has been expecting her. He has already calculated her due date from the wedding announcement he received three months earlier. It seems that he knew she was pregnant before she did.

In the ensuing discussion, her sensitive and innocent feminine nature and the doctor's professional authority are both emphasized. This patient is the exemplar of the nicely domestic woman, newly married and now preparing for motherhood. She objects to the "rabbit test" because the rabbit has to die: "'The poor thing! I wouldn't want to do that. . . . Couldn't you use a rat?'" (#11 194). He responds reassuringly: "'You'd better leave that to me'" (194). At the end of the exam, the patient is excited and eager to see an X-ray of the child. "'What a thought—having a picture of one's baby before it was born! I'm so interested in all this'" (194). Doctor Safford responds: "'I see that you are and I approve of it'" (194).

A very notable characteristic of this series is that all of the stories are cliffhangers. Just as the doctor has diagnosed the woman's problem, the case history ends with "To Be Continued." We leave one poor woman on her way to the hospital for a biopsy on a lump in her breast with a possible related endometrial problem (#10 31). Certainly, this kind of suspense makes for good magazine sales as most readers will fret over the fate of the women, not only because they have become interested but also because the very same problems may happen to them. Overall, these cases are very informative for the reader, but they are also rather judgmental and possibly frightening. Safford has done an excellent job of reinforcing the need for medical expertise, infusing his message with his own moral stance on such issues as abortion, sexually transmitted diseases, and artificial insemination.

When these "Tell Me Doctor" accounts appeared in 1950, *Ladies's Home Journal* had already been in publication for 67 years. Though not all of the women's magazines that began in the nineteenth century have survived into the twentieth, those that have survived create a solid foundation for the industry, bringing much of their nineteenth-century heritage with them. Of the "seven sister" publications in the women's service magazine category, three have been in publication for over 100 years: *McCall's* (1870), *Ladies' Home Journal* (1883), and *Good Housekeeping* (1885) (Wood 103, 105). The remaining four have been in publication since the first half of the twentieth century: *Redbook* (1903), *Better Homes & Gardens* (1922), *Family Circle* (1932), and *Woman's Day* (1938) (Garvey 674, Wood 337, 264, 259). The seven sisters have a combined circulation of over 30 million (Katz and Katz 1066). Since the industry standard is to multiply the number of subscribers by three to determine the number of actual readers for each magazine, we can assume that these seven publications are reaching approximately 90 million. The four "little sisters"—the fashion magazines *Glamour*, *Vogue*, *Cosmopolitan*, and *Mademoiselle*—add another 22.5 million readers to this audience (Redbook Research) for a total of 112.5 million. For the sake of comparison, monthly commentary magazines such as *Ms.* and *The New Republic*, which traditionally invite and publish critical commentary on a variety of topics, have approximate circulations of 466,154 and 45,000 respectively (Katz and Katz 1073, 815).

The primary research for this study includes 91 articles on the topic of assisted reproduction that were printed in the seven women's service magazines, four fashion magazines, and two weekly women's magazines over a period of twenty-one years: 1977 to 1997. Of these articles, 56, or 62%, are case histories narrating the stories of women who have received treatment for infertility. Of the 56 that tell stories, 50, or 89%, are positive accounts of the experience. Ironically, this fictitious 89% success rate is nearly the opposite of the average reported success rate for fertility treatment of 12% (Neumann, Gharib, and Weinstein 241). Magazines that are particularly likely to give potential fertility customers a skewed view of the efficacy of treatment include the three oldest: *Good Housekeeping* (*GH*), *Ladies' Home Journal* (*LHJ*), and *McCall's*. *LHJ* has the distinction of having printed the most articles on the topic: 17; the most cases: 16; and, to date, it is the only one of the seven sisters that has not published a critique of the fertility industry.

The following selected profiles should provide a better understanding of the women's service magazine's history and philosophy. At the ripe old age of 115 and with a circulation of 4.1 million (Katz and Katz 1071), *LHJ* is one of the standard bearers in the industry. The *Journal* had a colorful beginning with Edward Bok at its helm. His exposé of the patent medicine manufacturers contributed significantly to the passage of the Food and Drug Act (Wood 117) and his 1906 campaign to educate his readers about venereal disease brought lifesaving information to many women, despite the lost circulation and the criticism it provoked (119).

We have seen examples of *LHJ*'s promotion of domesticity in the 1950s; it now covers "parenting, family life, and women's changing roles . . . . *LHJ* believes that women today are living on a dual track, and [it] appears to be reaching for an updated, intelligible philosophy" (Katz and Katz 1071). *LHJ* continues to promote domesticity, albeit an updated version. The typical reader has a high school education and her average age is 44 (Redbook Research).

Founded in 1885, just two years after *LHJ*, *Good Housekeeping* has been sending its 5.2 million readers the same messages about domesticity for 113 years (Katz and Katz 1070). The magazine's editorial goal is "'to uphold high levels of good taste'" (qtd. in Katz and Katz 1070) and its articles are largely based on nostalgia or personal accounts (1070). Written for a general audience with an average age of 43, it also has a significant number of readers in the over 50 group (Redbook Research).

Like the *Journal*, *Good Housekeeping*'s nineteenth-century accomplishments were considerable. The Good Housekeeping Institute provided information on the quality of household merchandise and grew into a sophisticated laboratory that did its own testing prior to affixing its coveted "Good Housekeeping Seal" on those products that passed its scrutiny (Wood 123).

Since many of the readers of these two journals are in their fifties, until recently they have not been a direct market for reproductive technologies. These demographics are supported by the advertisements that surround the case histories. Along with the usual ads for feminine products, clothing, foods, recipes, and makeup, we find arthritis medicine, Oil of Olay for the woman whose daughter just went off to college, and grandma trading an Etch-A-Sketch for a hug. This older reader is, however, quite likely to have daughters, which makes her an important secondary audience. The advertisements may not appeal to her directly, but she will certainly think of a daughter in pain as she reads Laurie Steel's tale of barren woe in *Good Housekeeping*. The advertisement for Gerber baby food that has been placed there will only make the problem more poignant.

While reading about Louise Richards' four surrogacies in *LHJ*, our grandmotherly type will probably not consider buying the item advertised on the opposing pages for her childless daughter. "Bundle of Joy" is "an enchanting porcelain doll capturing all the warmth and innocence of a newborn baby" (23), complete with its own hospital I.D. bracelet. On the other hand, our reader can now tell her daughter where to go for help since Richards' story gives the name of the agency: Surrogate Parenting in Louisville, Kentucky. Having her mothers' support may be a crucial factor for the young woman considering reproductive technology.

The Oil of Olay advertisement that appears on the second page of the Journal's exclusive coverage of the Leslie Brown story is a subtle reminder of the potential influence of this older audience. "Isabel," who is now using Oil of Olay to preserve her looks, has recommended it to her daughter. The two confide in each other. The daughter, who is now also a good friend, follows her mother's advice (64). When Isabel's daughter is ready to start a family, she may need the assistance of reproductive technology and she will probably want her mother's approval. After reading the heartwarming birth stories printed in the pages of her trusted magazine, her mother will be much more disposed to grant it. Titles in *LHJ* read like a menu of available repro-tech services: "I Had My Sister's Baby," "Giving the Gift of Life," "Brave New Baby," and "Our Miracle Daughter." The women depicted in these stories are exemplary illustrations of *LHJ*'s motto: "Never Underestimate the Power of a Woman." *Good Housekeeping* can match the *Journal*'s coverage tear for tear, personal story for personal story. Indeed, *GH* appears to have affixed its prized seal on the procedures without the benefit of the scientific testing to which it submits other household products. The emotional first person accounts, with titles like "Kim Casali's Miracle Baby," "God Willed It," and "*Good Housekeeping* Gave Us Our Son," make the magazine's endorsement of modern technology as apparent as the value it places on motherhood.

Appealing to a younger audience of fashion, beauty, and health conscious women, *Redbook* and *Glamour* have lower circulations than their older counterparts—and racier editorial policies. They also offer a more balanced presentation of reproductive technology than *LHJ* and *GH*. *Redbook*, though considered one of the seven sisters, blurs the lines between the service and fashion categories for its 3.3 million readers (*Redbook* Research). Boasting that it is an editorial rebel by virtue of its greater coverage of beauty and fashion issues (*Redbook* Research), the magazine prefers articles that "entertain, educate, and inspire [its] readers to confront challenging issues" (Garvey 674). Katz and Katz characterize its tone as "confident, even brash" and say that it "pulls no punches" on matters of sexuality (1074). To its credit, of its 14 articles on reproductive technology, four are commentaries that examine the issues raised by such practices as egg donation and sperm banking and two of the cases were written by surrogate mothers who now disapprove of the practice. Overall, the coverage afforded to reproductive technology provided by *Redbook* is fairly balanced, presenting both critical and positive views of its value.

Glamour was founded in 1939 and has a circulation of 2.3 million (Garvey 670). This glossy fashion magazine is responsible for printing perhaps the best critical article on reproductive technology in any of the traditional women's magazines. Sociologist Barbara Katz Rothman is a professor at CUNY and she has written a book on the topic, *Recreating Motherhood*. Sandwiched between an eight-page spread of very young, very thin bathing suit models, and a seven-page spread of equally young, equally gorgeous hair and makeup models, "The Frightening Future of Baby-Making" is a surprise find in these pages. And it is not the only critical article *Glamour* has published. In 1989, Rasa Gustaitis' exposé of what she calls "Infertility Hype" warns readers to choose their fertility specialists carefully. This exposé is balanced by a defense of surrogacy written in 1991 by one of *Glamour*'s contributing editors. Another small article also printed in 1991 profiles a lesbian woman who fought for and lost visitation rights to two children her former partner gave birth to through artificial insemination. However, the editors do insult their readers by stamping the word controversy in big block letters across the page of this article. So *Glamour* too presents a rather mixed bag where coverage of reproductive technology is concerned.

Woman's World (*WW*) and *First For Women* (*FFW*) could be considered to be at the "low-brow" end of the women's magazine industry. Published weekly rather than monthly, both are recent entries into the market: *Woman's World* in 1981 and *First For Women* in 1989 (Katz and Katz 1077, Ulrich's 2753). With circulations of about 1.5 million both magazines reach a smaller audience than their bigger sisters (Katz and Katz 1077, Ulrich's 2753).

Though *WW* invites articles that cover "controversial, dramatic, and human interest women's issues," (Garvey 675) the controversy seems entirely left out of its pages. Katz and Katz describe the magazine as busy and cluttered and find value only in the food section. "*Woman's World* covers just about everything briefly and not very well. It is an exercise in oversimplification" (1077). With articles on losing weight, child safety, adoption, children with cancer, how to strengthen your marriage, and home furnishings, and a child on almost every page, it is easy to see that this magazine is aimed at the young mother. It comes as no surprise then to find the story of Kim Arnott's miracle babies (quadruplets) on the cover of one issue, and Naomi Durst's bouncing quadruplets on another.

First For Women has not been in publication long enough for Katz and Katz to have passed judgment on it, but with the same publisher as *WW*, its format is strikingly familiar. (The quality of the paper and the layout are better.) Like its sister publication, its best offerings are in the food section. It also has home, family, and health articles aimed at the young mother. Every issue has a story on childbirth and its most striking case history is illustrated by a cover photo of soap opera actress Deidre Hall holding her "miracle baby" born with the help of a contract mother.

The stories told in these women's magazines almost always relate happy endings, deflecting reality in favor of a highly sensational fantasy. This fantasy ideal is still based on the four qualities that defined the cult of true womanhood in the nineteenth century: purity, piety, domesticity, and submission. The case histories form a persuasive body of texts which demonstrates these four qualities in the "modern" mother and convinces the reader that reproductive technologies make it possible to attain them through the medical miracle: "[I]t was a miracle of modern medicine" (Baker 46); "She is a miracle" (Remsberg 73); "We've shared the miracle of life" (Richards 22); "Sam's birth . . . was literally a medical miracle" (Edmondson Gupta 141); Arlette Schweitzer "tells her miraculous story" (Schweitzer and Casey 125); and finally, "Our Miracle Daughter" (Travaglini 24).

Using Burke's pentadic relationships, the narrator of the case history in the women's magazine can be defined as the agent who narrates her story. The scene is then defined very narrowly as the case itself. This analysis will focus on the pentadic definitions that result from narrowing the interpretation of scene in this manner. Doing so allows a detailed look at the relationships between the author/narrator, the text she creates, and the sister reader who becomes her audience. Knowing how the reader of the women's magazine is constructed textually is crucial to understanding how women become willing participants in experimental technologies. When the scene is interpreted as the case history, the agent can then be defined as the new mother whose purpose is both to proclaim her newfound status as a legitimate mother and to justify the costly and painful means to her end. She does this through the act of constructing a sensationalized narrative of her techno-sex experience for her sister reader—an act which also becomes an endorsement of reproductive technologies.

Of particular interest is the agency or means by which the writer of the case history accomplishes the glorification of the techno-sex experience. This agency is the narrative structure shared by the case histories examined for this study—a rich hybrid of cultural genres comprised of elements of the fairy-tale, heroic quest, and religious miracle. Because this hybrid narrative structure draws on values and myths that are embedded in our culture, it is a highly effective tool for accomplishing the agent's purpose. The narrative structure allows the woman who participates in reproductive technologies to minimize—for herself and her reader—the physical and mental costs of attaining motherhood through assisted reproduction. At the same time, she sends the message to her reader that her ability to endure such hardships is the mark of the true woman's desire to reproduce. She sets a new standard for the "normal" woman, even as she argues that she is no different from the woman who has achieved motherhood in the old-fashioned way. Her quest also implies that without children, women cannot be complete. To reinforce the degree to which the narrator appears to have control over her journey to self-fulfillment, the medical technology she makes use of is portrayed as a powerful transforming device which she herself has invoked. The wand of technology is a potent tool, its narrative roots growing from both alchemy and religion. The doctor who wields the wand is characterized as a benevolent, grandfatherly Merlin, devoid of any of the basest of human motivations. Greed, ambition, pride, and conceit are completely edited from his character. He is often depicted as the right hand of God, collaborating with his maker in the very creation of life. Finally, the baby, or mythic boon, is always described as a perfect cherub, an angel sent from heaven. Quadruplets and quintuplets are photographed stretched serenely along their mothers' all-inclusive arms, smiling at the camera, the picture of health, the months they spent in intensive neonatal care written into the fine print of the story.

Within the pages of the women's magazine, the narrator/agent of the case history tells her story in a variety of ways. Most often, she writes her own story, giving a first person account of her emotional journey to motherhood. Alternatively, she tells her story to a professional writer who functions as a more literate scribe. Less common are articles in which the woman's experience is related through quotes selected by a professional author who takes control of the story. Despite the differing methods for telling these stories, the narrative characteristics remain remarkably constant, and the woman who tells of her experience with reproductive technology appears to have authority over the construction of her experience. This authority is complicated however, by her portrayal of herself as the heroine of her fairy-tale. By assigning herself a role within the narrative structure of the story, she redefines herself as an element of the agency as well.

To accomplish her purpose of legitimizing her status as a mother, the narrator draws on the archetypal characteristics of the fairy-tale heroine. She presents herself not as royalty, but as an ordinary, suffering woman, more akin to Cinderella than to Sleeping Beauty, waiting for childbirth to rescue her from the cinders of childlessness and make her complete. "Who cares about me? I'm a nobody from Plattsburg, N.Y.," (135), says Doris Del Zio. Leslie Brown tells the world, "'we're just two ordinary people with a simple ordinary name. We're the Browns'" (qtd. in Libman Block 71). Laurie Steel transforms herself into Cinderella-at-the-ball by dressing in a magical velvet gown. She wears this garb into Dr. Steptoe's operating room, hoping fervently that his magic wand will make the transformation permanent: "A tradition has developed among the women at Bourn Hall to dress for the occasion [implantation]. Laurie brushed her long blond hair, [and] put on makeup and a magenta velvet gown" (Remsberg 106).

The fairy-tale heroine is also capable of enduring all physical obstacles preventing her from accomplishing her goal. Pain, inseparable from childbearing for as long as humanity can remember, is an expected characteristic of motherhood, but technological motherhood includes suffering inconceivable even to Eve in the midst of her worst labor pains. An example of the case history heroine's physical commitment to motherhood is evident in Leslie Brown's willingness to allow Dr. Steptoe to remove her fallopian tubes because they were "in the way" of the procedures he wanted to perform:

> Nothing slowed Leslie. Uncomplaining, she underwent dozens of tests and explorations. She permitted Dr. Steptoe to completely remove her *useless* Fallopian tubes. The operation was extremely painful and on the long train ride back to Bristol from Oldham the wound in her stomach began to bleed. Leslie was in agony until she reached home and John could gently pull away the layers of her clothes that had become glued to her by her clotting blood. [emphasis added] (Libman Block 66)

Doris Del Zio's description of her physical condition after three operations to open her blocked fallopian tubes is equally gruesome: "My abdomen now looked like a road map and my insides were a mass of adhesions. Sometimes they were so painful that I just couldn't straighten up" (200). Arlette Schweitzer testifies that to achieve her goal (bearing twins for her daughter), "'I think [I] could even walk on coals if [I] had to'" (qtd. in Nash 58). Laurie Steele's perky reaction to hearing about Steptoe's in vitro work sums up the new standard for motherly commitment: "'I don't mind being a guinea pig'" (qtd. in Remsberg 105).

The mythical quest, a feature of the agency of the case history, adds another strategy for legitimizing the techno-mom's position: emphasizing the requisite characteristic of perseverance. Using the language of the fairy-tale, freelance writer Bonnie Remsberg describes Laurie Steel as "a long-legged, suntanned California blonde, bursting with good health and honest charm" (75). Despite a medical condition that prevented pregnancy, Steel tried to conceive for twelve years because she "simply, instinctively and profoundly wanted to have a baby, to love it, to meet the challenge of raising it, and to share it with Jon" (Steel qtd. in Remsberg 75).

In another account that emphasizes the normalcy of this type of odyssean tenacity, Claudia Franson tells her reader: "'I don't think I was fanatical about having a baby. I just didn't want to give up without having tried everything'" (qtd. in Baker 50). "Everything" amounted to a seven-year quest. She took Clomid (a powerful hormone that stimulates ovulation), had surgery to remove an adhesion, was treated for a microscopic infection, and miscarried. Yet despite all of these impediments, shortly after the birth of a son, she and her husband were already preparing to try to conceive a second time.

Soap opera actress Deidre Hall's quest for motherhood took her twenty years and three husbands. Like the others, she subjected herself to the entire gamut of fertility treatments:

> "I injected myself with hormones, tried artificial insemination and had every hand in the medical profession up my skirt trying to figure out what was wrong with me." (qtd. in Radovsky 37)

Hall's "20-year struggle for son David" (Radovsky 37) is profiled in the newer and less substantial women's magazine, *First For Women*, but after the birth of her second son (compliments of the same genetic/gestational mother), she tells her story of "What We Did for Love" in *LHJ* (Hall). In an opening line that sends a disturbing message about the "appropriate" role of the 90's woman, Hall explains how her life is now completely fulfilled as a result of her social motherhood:

> I used to be a driven person, one of the baby boomers who live from goal to goal. But ever since I became a mother, that ambition has completely fallen away. Now I can't wait to rush home from work and hug my sons David, three, and Tully, who turns one next month. (Hall 74)

By writing herself as a suffering fairy-tale heroine, on an heroic quest for the ultimate feminine fulfillment, the narrator of the case history achieves two objectives. The first is that she accomplishes her purpose of legitimizing her status as a mother. The second is perhaps not intentional; she has revised for her reader the definitions of some key characteristics of motherhood. Because she depicts herself as a heroine who begins as an ordinary woman desiring motherhood, she sets new standards for those ordinary women who make up her readership. The modern woman must show her commitment to motherhood by adding reproductive technologies to her repertoire of strategies for achieving her goal. Adding reproductive technologies means raising her capacity for physical endurance, pursuing her goal beyond all physical, emotional, and financial boundaries, and intensifying her belief that motherhood is the ultimate feminine achievement. Through the indoctrination provided by the case history, these new extremes have been rationalized and normalized for the next generation of women.

No fairy tale is complete without magic, and in the case history the wand of reproductive technology draws its power from magic and miracle. The doctor/facilitator who waves it is a benevolent Merlin figure and God's creative colleague; his altruistic crusade to coax new lives into the world has God's full blessing. In her dual role as narrator/agent and heroine/agency, the narrator both summons/prays for the magical miracle of reproductive technology and submits to and is transformed by it. Steptoe is depicted as the kindly grandfather of the technology. He is described in Leslie Brown's story as a "brilliant gynecologist" (Libman Block 64). For Laurie Steel, he is the "genial, gray-haired doctor" (Remsberg 105), "deeply devoted to the reproductive health and well-being of women" (104). Steptoe's more contemporary colleagues now appear in the women's magazine as expert advisors, warning the reader that if she is over 38, she should not try to reproduce without medical assistance (McDowell 31). The names and locations of the fertility clinics operated by these helpful advisors are also conveniently provided.

Perhaps the most compelling combination of the benevolent doctor working medical miracles through the magical powers of technology is contained in Remsberg's narration of Steel's implantation by Steptoe. Steel represents the Cinderella character: she dresses in a flowing magenta gown and prepares her hair and make-up in anticipation of the act of techno-sex in which she is about to participate. Entering the operating room at night because Steptoe likes to perform the procedure "when the uterus is quiet" (Remsberg 106), she waits while the embryo is carried in from the laboratory. Steptoe takes the long tube that encases it—the wand of technology—and "places it through the cervix into the womb. He waits several minutes, then removes the instrument" (108). Magical doctor, phallic technology, miraculous transformation: it comes as no surprise to read that "when the procedure was over, Laurie felt hugely relieved" (108).

Children, once considered gifts from God, are now miraculous GIFTs (gamete intrafallopian tube transfers) from the fertility clinic. If God has willed that a technology be created, then the aspiring mother is obliged to participate in it. Doris Del Zio explains: “I’m firmly convinced that there is a bond between science and religion. I always say a prayer for my doctor before I undergo surgery” (200). Leslie Brown “‘reckoned that God wanted [her] to have this baby or He wouldn’t have let that miracle of modern science happen to [her]’” (qtd. in Libman Block 67). “Dick” and “Cynthia,” the first ZIFT (zygote intrafallopian tube transfer) parents make a similar connection: “‘Why would God have created the technology that made ZIFT surrogacy possible if He didn’t want people to use it?’” (qtd. in Edmondson Gupta 216). Arlette Schweitzer had a more difficult religious dilemma because she is a “devout Catholic” and her church opposes surrogacy (189). She put her problem into “God’s hands” (189). As a sort of double affirmation of her faith in both God and science, she carried twins. A more recent ethical/moral dilemma occurs when reproductive technology produces multiple fetuses and women and their partners are faced with what one critical author calls the “Sophie’s Choice of selective reduction”—deciding whether to “reduce” the pregnancy by aborting some of the fetuses (Eberlein 89). In this situation, many women have tried so long and so hard to conceive that the idea of aborting any of the fetuses is unthinkable. Those with strong religious beliefs find themselves on new moral boundaries and many—like the newest media celebrities Bobby and Kenny McCaughey—fall back on their faith to answer such questions. One mother explains to her readers: “Because of our religious beliefs, Steve and I wouldn’t consider it [reduction]. . . . Fortunately, my faith got me through. I kept thinking God had brought us this far and that he’d continue to take care of us” (Clifford 56). When God’s support is invoked in this way, the ethical issues can be pushed to the side, while the aspiring mother’s dedication and tenacity are forefronted.

If the doctor plays the magician in these technological tales, then the role of the fairy godmother goes to the woman who plays the role of surrogate mother. She contributes to the agency of the narrative structure by facilitating the happiness of the narrator/agent—just as Cinderella’s fairy godmother helped her to attend the ball. Her magic lies in her ability to conceive: “‘I have babies so easily—they just pop out’” (Kane qtd. in Markoutsas 98). The use of the term surrogate implies that she is not really a mother at all, but a "human incubator" (qtd. in Edmondson Gupta 141).

Because she is depicted as so far removed from the physical act in which she is participating, the woman who contracts out her motherhood is made over into a safe character in the case history. This fairy godmother waves a magic linguistic wand that minimizes her relationship with the child she is carrying. For Karen Mills (1985), who was acting as a "traditional" surrogate (i.e.: supplying the egg and the womb), her baby was simply her "little passenger" while she was the "carrier" (209). "Debbie" says she was "'just a baby-sitter'" (qtd. in Edmondson Gupta 215). The women claim to bond instead with the aspiring mothers who are their clients. "Kathy," who says she "'had no emotional trouble giving up . . . twins,'" explains that her real bond is with the woman for whom she carried them (qtd. in Edmiston 237). Deidre Hall is proud of the fact that she and "Robin," who is both the genetic and gestational mother of Hall's children, bonded in what she calls a "'girlfriend process'" (qtd. in Radovsky 38). Hall even believes that "'having a child through a surrogate mother is more involving than having it come from your body, because you're forming a kinship with another woman as intimately as you can'" (38).

Sometimes that bond is biological, as in a recent case in which a 48 year-old woman conceived quadruplets using her 28 year-old sister's donated eggs. Despite having her own reproductive problems that may have been aggravated by the hormones she would have to use, the sister was eager to help: "Heidi told us that she was very honored that we'd thought of her, then listened closely as we described the risks. . . . The *small risk of ovarian cancer* still made Steve and me apprehensive, but Heidi was so anxious to help us that her enthusiasm eased our fears" (emphasis added Clifford 54). The surrogate/godmother's role also receives God's blessing in the case history: "Elizabeth Kane is a saint" (Markoutsas 96); another nameless birth mother is "a crusader" (98), and Hall believes that Robin "'came from God with [her] name on her'" (qtd. in Radovsky 37).

When surrogate mothers—genetic or gestational—refuse to honor the terms of their contracts, their narrative roles are easily rewritten. Because she has purchased the surrogate's services, the narrator uses her authorial control to stake her emotional claim to the child by transforming the fairy godmother into the wicked witch. The best illustration of how the wicked witch image is used to reassure aspiring mothers in the case history is the highly publicized custody suit that was fought over Baby M. This battle made Mary Beth Whitehead-Gould, the child's genetic and gestational mother, the most famous "surrogate" mother since that other Mary gave birth in a stable 1,998 years ago. Whitehead-Gould has become a mythic presence in the case history fairy-tale: the personification of the selfish woman who went back on her promise to deliver up her child to an unfulfilled aspiring mother. Her depiction by the justice system as a bad mother complicates more than the legal definition of motherhood. Characterized by the courts as an obsession, her desire to keep her child was considered evidence of her unfit status. Thus, her mothering instinct was used against her. Ironically, the only way she could have reversed this negative characterization was to agree to give up her child. The Baby M case helped to establish a split definition of the good mother in the case history. When a contract has been drawn up, the accepted nurturing role of the genetic and/or gestational mother begins and ends with supplying the genetic material and/or incubation necessary to create the child. Once that is accomplished, only the social mother is expected and allowed to nurture the child emotionally.

While the custody case was being fought, Whitehead-Gould did receive the opportunity to operate as agent and tell her story in the women's magazine. Excerpts from her book were printed in *Family Circle*. However, a 1994 profile in *Redbook* portrays her as an obsessive mother (Squire 96–98). Case histories in the last ten years are saturated with references to her as the negative example against which all potentially problematic women are measured. Readers are reassured when they discover that Robin, the woman hired by Deidre Hall to give birth, showed the film made about Baby M to her children to convince them that, unlike the bad woman in the movie, she would be doing a good deed by giving their sibling away (McDowell 38). A 1995 narrative reaffirms that Whitehead's symbolic "wicked witch" status remains unchallenged: "Mary Beth Whitehead single-handedly poisoned the pot" (Bransford 177).

When a mythic hero endures considerable suffering on a protracted odyssey, it is usually to gain a boon so great that even the risk of death is worth the reward. As the final element of the fairy tale/myth/miracle narrative structure of the case history, the baby has to be represented as the ultimate boon in order to fulfill this crucial position. For her role in the agency, the baby is both mythic holy grail and the angelic manifestation of God's will. The births are reported in the hyperbolic miracle language that has become the standard for the popular media: "She is a miracle" (Remsberg, 1982); "Our miracle daughter" (Travaglini, 1992); and "I'm living with a miracle" (Uchytil, 1993). They are also always described as perfect. Louise Joy Brown is a "cooing, gurgling, blue-eyed beauty" (Libman Block, 1979 62). Laurie Steel's Samantha is "a beautiful baby . . . gorgeously healthy and rosy looking (Remsberg, 1982, 108), and little Brent was born "healthy and robust, loudly protesting his rough introduction to life" (Baker, 1980 46).

If one child is a boon, then multiple births must be depicted as multiple blessings. The heroine of the case history becomes truly epic if she faces the challenge of mothering a large group of same-age children. She has returned from her torturous journey with not one holy grail but four or five. In articles with titles like "Love (times) 5" (Fein 96), "The Triplets Club" (Rock 144), "A Quint-essential Christmas" (Williams 107), "Oh baby, baby, baby, baby!" (Davenport 82), "God Gave Us Four Miracles" (Clifford 52), and "Cuter by the Half-Dozen" (Dilley 1998), the narrator/agent offers her sage advice to her sister readers who may be following her quest. Donations seem to pour in and neighborhoods rally around the new parents. No one sleeps much but no one seems to mind. Cheryl Clifford sums her view of quadruplet motherhood up in a catchy heading: "Marathon nights, assembly-line days—and no regrets whatsoever" (57).

The narrator/agent of the case history uses her account of the pain she experiences to legitimize herself as a mother. In so doing, she glosses over the multiple costs of participating in reproductive experimentation. Most women who participate in these experiments do not go home with babies. For them, the physical price has no final, fulfilling purpose. And the pain is quite real and intense. Janice Raymond considers egg "harvesting" to be medical rape:

> In the 1980s, an Austrian female student-observer described the vaginal harvesting of eggs from a woman in full view of a medical school class: "At each follicle puncture he [the doctor] retracted the needle and then drove it in hard. The woman asked him to stop, because she was in great pain. But Dr. M. would have none of that . . . and so [more] follicles were punctured against her will . . . again each puncture unmistakably resembled a penetration." (Raymond 32)

Reproductive technologies exact costs that go far beyond the physical pain they produce. People spend their savings, mortgage their homes, and go deeply into debt to finance their extravagant quests. The average reader of the women's magazine has an annual income of only $40,000 and the least expensive IVF baby is $67,000 (Neumann et al. 242). If the treatments are successful, there is a 50% chance that the pregnancy will be a multiple one, adding to the cost of care, delivery, and maintenance. Most women, however, will go home empty-handed and feeling as though they have failed to achieve the most important goal of their gender: motherhood.

For all of the women profiled here, there is a hierarchy of methods for attaining motherhood. The highest level of achievement is to bear a child genetically related to both aspiring parents. The next preference is to experience pregnancy and childbirth, even if this means the woman has to use an egg "donor." If this option is not possible, a woman is hired to carry a child created from the aspiring parents' genetic material; this option is followed by hiring a woman who "donates" her own egg and is fertilized with the contracting male's sperm. Finally, the last method on the list is adoption. For those who demand a biological connection, this solution is not considered an option, but for those who do choose it, adoption does not appear to be as fulfilling as pregnancy and childbirth, nor does it seem to qualify the woman as a "true" mother. Thus, even though a woman has children in her life, her own but not her present husband's, his from a previous marriage, or adoptive children, if she has the opportunity to acquire a child even remotely biologically connected to her or her mate and/or she can gestate herself, she must do so to properly consider herself a mother. The more actively she quests for control over the act of creation, the closer to "true" motherhood she comes. The testimony of one woman who used an egg donor implies a work ethic: "I've gone through more than most women would go through to give this baby life. If you think of it that way, it's more mine than anyone else's, because I had to work at it more" (Simon, qtd. in Liebman-Smith 178). Another's dedication to her struggle makes her feel almost God-like: "I fought so hard to have this baby that I feel ninety-nine-point-nine percent the creator" (Finlay, qtd. in Liebman-Smith 178). Ironically, that control is an illusion; in the fertility clinic, the manipulation of gametes is firmly in the hands of the medical practitioners, not the women who present themselves as research subjects.

Many of the women discussed here already had other children. Brown considered raising her step-daughter to be practice for the real thing (Libman Block 65). Del Zio had a biological daughter, but wanted a child with her present husband (135). Mills had already adopted a "Korean girl" (20), but she thinks the "sun rises and sets on Jessica," the baby her sister bore for her (190). Linda and Glenn Merkel had a child fathered by him with a surrogate, but when they heard that they could have a child genetically related to both of them, they decided to "'try something a little more challenging'" and hire a woman to gestate their embryo (G. Merkel qtd. in Edmiston. 236). Finally, "Elaina" and her husband "Sam" had already adopted two children, but when she had the opportunity to gestate a child with an egg donated by her best friend "Beth," she leapt at the chance: "In the labor room, all I did was cry, because I wanted the baby to be born, but I didn't want the pregnancy to end. I had had such a beautiful nine months—I had never felt so good in my life" (qtd. in Liebmann-Smith 177).

Pushed to the margins in these stories are the existing children, step, adoptive, and biological children with the "wrong" fathers or mothers. As they watch the nurturing women in their lives make the grueling journey to "genuine" motherhood, they must wonder about their own legitimacy. If their mothers are not already true mothers, then how can they be true sons and daughters? Placing a hierarchy on motherhood places the same hierarchical values on childhood.

Hall's story illustrates well the drive to accomplish motherhood regardless of the obstacles. Present at the birth of David, Hall seems to be unaware of the extreme nature of her desire to take possession of this child. She describes her actions in the delivery room: "As David came out I grabbed him, while Robin was saying, 'Take it easy!' He's still attached to me!' It was all so magical" (qtd. in Radovsky 38). Hall is not the only aspiring mother to nearly rip the baby from the womb of the woman she has hired to gestate for her. When Cynthia was allowed to hold her newly born son, "'she was ready to bundle him up and walk away.'" The doctor had to call out "'Wait, he's still attached!'" (Edmondson Gupta 216).

These women seem to forget that the mothers who are delivering babies into their arms are human, vulnerable, and even necessary. During Robin's second pregnancy, Hall wishes for something physically impossible, she wants to somehow remove Robin from the picture, even while she gestates. "Robin and I went shopping, ate lunch together and developed a real friendship. That's not to say that it was emotionally easy all the time. Once, at a visit to the obstetrician, I thought, Gee, it sure would be nice if Robin would leave so I could be alone with my baby" (Hall 75).

Another woman, H. Bransford, whose passion for a child led her to hire a woman to act as a surrogate, demonstrates how completely she has divorced this woman from the fetuses she is carrying. She made the mistake of hiring a woman who was both overweight and a chain smoker, and when the twin pregnancy resulted in gestational diabetes, Bransford explains the problems in a "diary" account now available to her reader:

> She also has a minor infection, and worst of all, she's still smoking. Combined with diabetes, smoking can cause insufficient blood flow to the babies, premature separation of the placenta from the uterus (i.e. death), low birthweight, and complicated circulatory problems. Damn her for doing a half-assed job. (177)

The potential for harm to the woman carrying the children—death—warrants a parenthetical reference, while the potential problems for the babies are the clear focus of this woman's concern. Like Hall, Bransford also wishes she could just dispense with the hired womb, especially because she is doing such a lousy job; because she cannot, she writes the fetuses letters of apology for "picking such a lousy carrier" (Bransford 177). Neither Hall nor Bransford seems to recognize the detached way in which they view the two women who are risking their lives to create children for them.

Unfortunately, the rosy picture painted by the narrator of the fairy godmother/surrogate glosses over the fact that women who rent out their wombs usually have worldly reasons for doing so. An example of how well the case history works to obscure the problematic nature of such arrangements is Bransford's narrative of her experience with "Hope," the chain smoking woman she wishes she could fire half way through the job. In an early diary entry, she comments about the legal status of surrogacy: "The laws seem antediluvian, and the fear of creating a breeding class of women ludicrous" (Bransford 176). Yet Bransford tells her reader that Hope shares a cramped apartment with her mother, sister, and an assortment of children, and she earns $8,000 a year as a waitress (134). She lives below poverty level and is clearly engaging in surrogacy for the money. Bransford also reveals her class prejudice when she writes in a letter to the unborn fetuses, "Please know I'll do better by you when you come out. You won't have to breathe smoke, eat McDonald's, or *listen to county-music TV day and night* [emphais added]" (177). One could argue that cigarette smoking and even the high fat content of some McDonald's foods could be harmful to a fetus, but how could listening to country music harm the babies, unless the author believes that they will come to enjoy it and that this preference will be somehow detrimental. Despite her frustrations about Hope's unsuitability as a carrier (both physically and culturally), Bransford, incapable or unwilling to recognize the exploitative relationship she has participated in, still paints a happy ending: "Today Hope has a car, her debt is behind her, she has an expanded support system, and she plans to attend paralegal school" (178).

When Doris Del Zio's fertilized eggs were destroyed by a doctor who did not agree with the ethics of the procedure, she accused him of playing God (202). What she and her sister questers seem to have missed is that the doctors who facilitate their reproduction can have less-than-altruistic motives. Financial gain and prestige are obvious draws to the fertility industry, but probably the most compelling motivation is that the fertility doctor gets to wave his magic wand over his patient and say, "Let there be life." Because human motivations are not addressed, the antics of doctors like Cecil Jacobson, who was accused of using his own sperm for inseminations, come as a shock to the trusting reader of the women's magazine. (Jacobson was fond of telling his patients: "God doesn't give you babies, I do") (qtd. in Elmer-DeWitt 27). A recent scandal involving the University of California at Irvine fertility clinic and Dr. Ricardo Asch, considered by the profession to be one of its leaders, has produced one case history in which the woman tells how she was betrayed by the doctor she trusted with her embryos (Challender 84). (Asch and two colleagues were accused of "stealing" embryos from patients) (Roberts 585). But such cases are rare in the women's magazine, and one need not read beyond the benevolent depiction of grandfatherly Dr. Steptoe to find questionable motives that have not been addressed. When Louise Joy Brown was delivered via a conveniently necessary cesarean section, her mother's missing fallopian tubes erased any doubt for observers that Steptoe had achieved in vitro fertilization. One wonders whether he removed them because they were in the way of his medical procedures or his reputation.

The babies edited out of these stories are those who arrive with birth defects. Instead the reader is introduced to the Arnotts' four little angels who were presumably sent from heaven to answer their prayers. In reality, the Arnotts' quadruplets arrived by cesarean section three months before term. Weighing in at between one and two pounds each, they spent the first three months of their lives in the neonatal unit at the hospital. The Arnotts were fortunate that their children have a 90% chance of developing normally (Simpson 13). Recalling the statistics cited in chapter one, babies that are the product of multiple birth pregnancies are usually born prematurely, with low birth weights, and they are far more susceptible to birth complications and defect. With multiple births on the rise, such problems are likely to become more and more common.

Edited into the margins along with birth defects are the financial and management costs of multiple births. The day-to-day lives of these families are presented as merely hectically humorous. When overwhelmed, the exhausted mothers simply "look back at being pregnant, worried and bedbound, and that puts it all into perspective" (Dunseith, qtd. in Rock 146). Faced with the kind of feminine heroism portrayed by these women, how can the reader refuse to include reproductive technology in her repertoire of strategies for achieving motherhood? To do less would be to fail as a woman.

In fact, after reading her daily fare of gynecological case histories over the past twenty years, the check-out stand reader has learned that to be a true woman she must have a child. She must be willing to pursue that child regardless of the costs—financial, physical, emotional, or social—to her, to the child, to her existing children, and to the women whose bodies she may have a hand in exploiting. She has learned that the doctors who perform these technological feats are benevolent wizards, whom she can and should trust with her reproductive power, that the technology is magical and potent, and that, if her quest demands it, other women's bodies and emotions are legitimately hers to exploit. The baby she may attain will not only be perfect, but it will bring her the ultimate feminine fulfillment: the completeness of motherhood. Finally, the entire journey is one that has been mandated by the will of God.

A modern version of the nineteenth-century cult of true womanhood saturates every rhetorical aspect of the case history in the women's service magazine. The emotional and highly subjective language of the first person narrative attracts the reader who, because she identifies with the storyteller, is more inclined to adopt the storyteller's unexamined belief in both motherhood at all costs and reproductive technology. This belief brings the childless woman into the fertility clinic and ensures her willing participation in a massive medical experiment that promises to change the way women reproduce, but not how they are valued in relation to reproduction. The redefinition of motherhood goes beyond reiterating and reproducing our existing "sexual caste system" (Daly 227); it adds a new hierarchy of classifications so that women may be valued according to their reproductive function: as social nurturers, as suppliers of genetic material, or as providers of gestational environments. The "ordinary" woman who purchases the women's service magazine and reads about these technologies must recognize how she is collaborating in the revision of feminine value. Whether or not her progeny is being genetically engineered in the laboratory, she is being linguistically engineered into this newly extended sexual caste system. Whether she occupies the more valued position of social nurturer or the low-ranking position of human incubator, as a member of the reproductive brothel she is participating in a continuing devaluation of women that is both dehumanizing and destructive—to her and to the society in which she lives.

Looking at the modern gynecological case history as a fairy tale means that many issues raised by the technology have either been left unaddressed or glossed over. In chapter four, "Gynecology on the Coffee Table," I will examine how the commentary magazines discuss the same technologies. These magazines refocus the discussion to consider their special concerns. The religious critic examines the God/science relationship. The feminist commentator considers the impact the technology has on the rights of women. The ethicist comments on the impact the scientific innovations will have on society, and those concerned with eugenics explore how the new technologies compare to other schemes to perfect the race. This kind of focused scrutiny renders impotent the fantasy depiction of reproductive technologies.

NOTES

1. Sanger attributes her "conversion" to the cause of birth control to her emotional reaction after witnessing the death of Sadie Sachs. Mrs. Sachs was a patient Sanger attended in New York's Lower East side. After nursing her back to health from one abortion attempt, Sanger was called back to the Sachs' home just a few months later to watch Sadie Sachs die (Kennedy 16). In his biography of Sanger, David Kennedy argues that she exaggerated her reaction to the incident in what he calls a "common autobiographical ploy of reformers" (17). Though he does not question her emotional reaction to Mrs. Sachs' death, he believes she used her account of the event to secure her status as a symbolic leader in the birth control movement.

CHAPTER FOUR

Gynecology on the Coffee Table

> What is new today is that conflicts reach the public through the courts and are being debated as individual cases, containing all the complexities and ambiguities of real life. . . . Because the issues are embedded in human stories, they are more gripping, and the debate is broader. That creates greater opportunity for widespread democratic opinion to be heard—and, of course, to be manipulated. (Gordon "Reproductive Rights" 230)

Writing for *The Nation* at the height of the Baby M trial, University of Wisconsin historian Linda Gordon gives this very appropriate analysis of the effect the litigious gynecological case history has had on national opinion. We have seen in chapter three how the case history can manipulate this opinion for one audience—the reader of the women's magazine. In that venue, the case history cuts off any productive debate by creating a fantasy of feminine fulfillment to promote new reproductive technologies. To find a debate that fully explores the complex issues created by these technologies, we must turn to the commentary magazines that are typically displayed on the coffee table of the educated middle-class reader. The commentary debate is limited, however, by the fact that, for the most part, the cases must make the news before they appear on the coffee table. As Gordon points out "the stories that reach us are of arrangements gone wrong" (230). For her this "soap-opera approach to reproductive conflicts obscures the social causes of all this litigation" (230). The happy endings profiled in the women's magazines obscure the many questions raised by reproductive technologies. The reactive nature of the commentary ensures a discussion but limits it to the specific issues that are raised by the problematic cases. Despite these limitations, the commentary discussion goes a long way towards debunking the myths created in the women's magazine.

Debunking myths comes naturally to the nation's commentary magazines. They are in the business of provoking debate. The commentary magazine depends upon an educated, up-to-date reader who appreciates a good moral, legal, or ethical argument. This change in scene brings a corresponding change in purpose: the modern gynecological case history now serves as a springboard for discussion. In the women's magazine, the case history was pressed into the service of that venue's promotion of motherhood. In the commentary journal, the case history can be appropriated for discussions focusing on concerns as diverse as women's rights, race and class relations, medical ethics, religious morality, and social policy. Voicing these concerns is a new and diverse set of agents. Whereas in the women's magazine the voice was for the most part homogenous, in the commentary magazine the voice becomes pluralistic; the feminist, the academic, the theologian, the medical ethicist, and the journalist are all found in these pages.

Because it is now only the instigator of the discussion, the case itself has a new agency. The focus is no longer on the personal story (though the personal is what brings the case to attention); the people whose lives are being debated fade to the background and come to represent the issues about which the intellectual discussion forms. Thus the Baby M case becomes significant not because it tells us about Mary Beth Whitehead's love for her daughter, but because it provokes a discussion of contract motherhood.

Like the lifestyles publication, the commentary magazine responded to the birth of Louise Joy Brown with a sharp increase in publications on reproductive technology. The commentary category is responsible for 147 articles, 16% of the 877 articles in the sample. To narrow the scope of my discussion, I have selected eight commentary journals based in part on their editorial policies and/or religious focus, and in part on the extent of their coverage of reproductive technology, or lack thereof. *The Nation*, *The New Republic*, *National Review*, and *Ms.* make up the secular group, and *Christian Century*, *Commonweal*, *America*, and *Commentary* represent the religious interests. Though library science categorizes *Ms.* as a lifestyles selection, I have added it to the commentary group because I think it is extremely out of place in the company of the decidedly traditional seven sisters. *Ms.* adds to the commentary discussion by raising a distinctly feminist voice.

Altogether, the seven commentary publications are responsible for 50 of the 147 commentary articles in the twenty years since the birth of Louise Joy Brown. *Ms.* adds another nine for a total sample of 59. Of these 59 articles, 30 are responses to specific case histories; over half of these—16—are reactions to the Baby M case. Six are arguments against cloning in response to the recent cloning of a sheep in Scotland, and just one addresses the birth of the McCaughey septuplets in November 1997. Nine of the authors are theologians and/or priests. Seventeen are academics. Thirty-one of the authors are men and seventeen are women—eight of whom are published in *Ms.* alone. The remaining articles are anonymous news pieces and editorials. In contrast to the contributors to the women's magazine, the authorship of the commentary journals is richly academic, greatly concerned with ethics, and decidedly masculine.

The circulations of these periodicals are difficult to compare with those of the women's magazines because many of the commentary journals are published weekly or bi-weekly rather than monthly. The weeklies have an approximate circulation of 218,000, the bi-weeklies 129,000, and the monthlies 511,000 (466,000 of this figure represents the readership of *Ms.* alone). Clearly, these publications have a far narrower audience than the 30 million total for the women's magazines. Because the commentary journals cater to specific political and/or religious viewpoints, the audiences of these publications tend to be more selective. While the reader of the women's magazine is quite likely to read more than one of the seven sisters, the readers of the commentary magazine, while sharing general characteristics such as education, may select only the one that reflects their specific orientation.

The Nation is the oldest journal in the sample. Established in 1865, it has a weekly circulation of 50,000 and is staunchly liberal (Katz and Katz 818). Katz and Katz praise its investigative reports and describe its editorials as "quite superior in both content and style" (818). A look at its advertising confirms that its audience, which ranges from those with a high school education to those in academia (818), is economically stable enough to be investing in both the future and PBS. The reader of *The Nation* is interested in investing in his/her mind. The majority of advertising is for books and literary videos.

Three of the four articles published on reproductive technology in *The Nation* were written in a three-year period beginning in May 1987 and ending in December 1990. The Baby M case was the main impetus for this coverage. The articles are substantial pieces written by women with impressive credentials. Two are by Katha Pollitt, an award winning poet, feminist critic, and frequent contributor to *The Nation*, who confirms the opinion that "[s]ome of the best stylists in journalism are regular columnists" in *The Nation* (Katz and Katz 818). The third is by Linda Gordon, the University of Wisconsin historian and author of a feminist history of birth control in America. The fourth is a recent article written by Columbia University law professor, Patricia J. Williams, in response to the cloning of Dolly the lamb in Scotland. *The Nation* has the distinction of being the only commentary journal in my sample, with the exception of *Ms.*, to publish only female authors on the topic.

Though it was established to be a liberal voice in 1914, *The New Republic* now attempts to take a balanced approach to its commentary. According to Katz and Katz, the *New Republic* prints "lively criticism . . . of the current political and economic scene. . . " (819), and "[t]he conservative as well as the voice of the left is heard in its pages" (819). The magazine publishes weekly and has a healthy circulation of 95,000.

The New Republic's seven offerings include two commentary pieces with the playful title "In Vitro Veritas." The editors obviously expect the reader to understand the pun and chuckle at the comparison between wine and "bottled babies," something an educated reader would do quite readily. Its advertising reflects its attempt to reach a politically diverse audience. PBS, financial planning, and books are highlighted, and a full-page argument for zero population growth is placed near a PR piece for a Northrop-Grumman bomber. Except for a recent piece by Michael J. Sandel, a professor of Political Science at Harvard, the commentary authors are journalists, with only one female co-author.

With a bi-weekly readership of 110,000, *National Review* has the highest circulation of the commentary publications (with the exception of *Ms.*) (Katz and Katz 818). Established in 1955 and edited by William F. Buckley, it is "[t]he premier conservative journal" publishing "on topics of current political, social and cultural interest" (818). The advertising in this publication reflects the conservative bent of its audience. Conservative summits and symposiums are offered, along with the now-common ads for financial planning, books (conservative), and Northrop-Grumman. PBS is absent.

National Review has six articles on reproductive technologies, but most are very brief reaction pieces. Of these six, the most substantial one is titled "Womb to Let." In response to the Whitehead custody case, the assistant article editor Maggie Gallagher makes a witty, yet forceful statement about the practice of surrogacy. It's a pity that *National Review* has not printed more on the subject.

Commentary, established in 1945, with a monthly circulation of 45,000, prints articles on matters of general political and cultural interest. A Jewish publication, its purpose is to "enlighten and clarify public opinion on problems of Jewish concern. . . ."(Katz and Katz 815). It comes as no surprise that its one article on reproductive technologies—albeit written by a Lutheran minister—is a warning that they will lead to a modern eugenics. Most of its advertising has some link to Middle Eastern issues.

Commonweal represents a liberal Catholic perspective on current issues. Established in 1924, it does not hesitate to challenge the Church when it disagrees with its policies or views (Katz and Katz 935). Since its advertising appears to target the lay Catholic rather than the clergy, perhaps this audience is more likely to tolerate some criticism of the Roman authority. With only 19,000 bi-weekly readers it has the smallest circulation of the group, but it has published the most articles on reproductive technology. Of its thirteen articles, three were written by women and six are editorials taking a firm stand against commercial surrogacy. Seven of the articles are responses to the Baby M case. The most recent article uses the McCaughey septuplets as a springboard for a critique of the ethical dilemmas created by multiple pregnancies.

The clerical counterpart to *Commonweal* is *America*; established in 1909 with a weekly circulation of 35,000, it is published by the Jesuits of the U.S. and Canada (Katz and Katz 933). The journal presents views on current issues: religious, political, social, and cultural (Katz and Katz 933). The market for parish census software probably does not extend beyond the rectory, and the many additional advertisements for seminary schools, the Army chaplain corps, and study seminars in Rome confirm that the audience is more likely to be pastor than parishioner.

The nine articles published in *America* also reflect its clerical audience. The first moves tediously through papal proclamations on artificial methods for reproduction, looking for but not finding a loophole big enough to permit them. Another defends a judge's decision that seven frozen embryos were indeed children and should be awarded to their genetic mother in a custody suit. A 1996 article by Robert J. White, professor of surgery at Case Western, responds to the destruction of 3300 embryos in Britain. He argues that embryos are fully human, materially and spiritually, and that they should be awarded full rights. The two most recent publications are reactions to the cloning of Dolly the lamb, one by Kevin T. Fitzgerald, a Jesuit priest who is also a molecular geneticist at Loyola University, and the other by Stephen G. Post, a bioethicist at Case Western Reserve University. Both make cases for banning human cloning.

Christian Century represents the Protestant point of view with articles that are "strong on ethical and social issues" and written for the educated layperson and religious professional (Katz and Katz 934). A moderate to liberal journal, it tries to take other religious views into account. In publication since 1908, the journal has a weekly circulation of 38,500 (934). Its advertising indicates the greater diversity of its audience: theological seminaries and insurance companies are offered along with Pastor Marty's recipes. The *Christian Century* has published thirteen articles on a variety of issues raised by the new technologies, its authors generally developing carefully reasoned arguments that grant a qualified acceptance of some of the basic reproductive technologies. A 1996 report on Cardinal Basil Hume's reaction to the British embryo purge breaks with that acceptance. Hume urges scientists to pursue other morally acceptable means for treating infertility so that the practice of creating and freezing embryos can be discontinued.

Ms. was established in 1972 to express feminist concerns and today it "stands fearless, willing to confront the controversies of the day that *Ms.* sees as continuing issues: motherhood in an age of reproductive choices and technology, child-care legislation, career discrimination, homeless women" (Katz and Katz 1073). Its monthly circulation of 466,154 shows that it has a far wider audience than any of the other commentary journals described here (1073). *Ms.* no longer runs advertisements in its pages because the editors felt the concerns of the advertisers were limiting the scope of their commentary. The journal is now supported entirely by subscriptions. All nine pieces discussing reproductive technology were written by women, and whether they support such practices or not, all take a close look at how they affect women.

Though the readers of the commentary magazines differ in their political viewpoints and religious convictions, they are all educated, critical readers who are interested in discussions of social and cultural problems. Even if they do read the version of the case history presented in the women's magazine, it is unlikely they will be drawn in by the fabulous pictures these cases create. The readership of the commentary journal will, however, be interested in the intellectual debate inspired by the case history in the commentary journal. This debate, ranging from the theological to the feminist, is far more likely to condemn modern reproductive practices. The commentators express concerns that the new technologies will violate women's rights and bodies; commodify women and children; disrupt the marriage relationship; devalue the sanctity of human life; lead us to a modern eugenics; and cause public policy nightmares. Though they are not expressed as direct responses to the representation of the case history found in the women's magazine, the commentators' concerns do address the belief-system that is intrinsic to that venue's fairy-tale representation. Examining how the components of the fairy-tale/myth presented in the women's magazine are treated in this more critical venue will show how the fable falls apart in the commentary discussion.

The first component of the fairy tale/myth is the questing mother whose pain and suffering were well worth the gain—the perfect baby. The problem with this view is that success rates for IVF procedures are actually quite low. Janice Raymond, professor of women's studies and medical ethics at University of Massachusetts, Amherst, writing for *Ms.*, claims that clinics skew their data by reporting statistics based on egg harvesting, implantation, and chemical pregnancy. None of these statistics means that a live birth has been achieved. Raymond reports that the "take-home baby rate" in the United States in 1991 was only nine percent (30).[1] A July 1994 study published in the *New England Journal of Medicine* quotes an average take-home baby rate of only 12% (Neumann, Soheyla, and Weinstein 241). This means that up to 88% of the women who go through these procedures will remain childless. These are the stories that are not being told in the women's magazine.

To make real the pain these women experience, Raymond's exposé brings us into the operating room to see a "vaginal harvesting" as it is being performed (32). The medical student's observation that an egg "retrieval" procedure bears a close resemblance to forced penetration—techno-rape—motivates Raymond to characterize reproductive technologies as "torture techniques" (28).

If this characterization seems to be the exaggeration of an angry feminist, it can be compared to testimony given in a *Redbook* portrait of a woman named Beth who donates eggs to her friend Elaina. Beth describes the egg retrieval procedure as "'the pits'" (qtd. in Liebmann-Smith 174).

> "I had to be in a weird position, lying with my legs strapped up real high and pushed back against my chest . . . . I was there from seven a.m. until four p.m. My hips were throbbing so much that, when I got home, I couldn't move or sleep all night" (174).

Though Beth dismisses this pain as "'irrelevant,'" emphasizing instead her pride that the eggs retrieved were all graded "'excellent to superior'" (174), her account confirms the point Raymond makes about the extreme pain the procedure incurs.

Even more worrisome is the fact that IVF procedures are experimental and potentially harmful to women's reproductive systems. A *Commonweal* editorial expresses concern over the fact that "[t]here was no groundwork of primate experimentation" prior to the experiment carried out on Leslie Brown's body ("Test-Tube Babies" 548). Raymond adds that chemical superovulation can lead to ovarian cysts and hyperstimulation. She tells the reader that at least ten deaths connected to IVF procedures have been documented (30).[2]

One of the most potent aspects of the women's magazine myth is that reproductive technologies enhance motherhood. Katha Pollitt, Linda Gordon, and Maggie Gallagher argue that contractual motherhood instead degrades motherhood by fragmenting its definition and equating pregnancy with sperm donation. In her noted essay on the Baby M case printed in *The Nation*, Pollitt contends that while men and women make equal genetic contributions, merely contributing genes is not sufficient to describe the woman's role in creating a child:

> [T]wenty-three pairs of chromosomes do not a baby make. In the usual course of events the woman is then pregnant for nine months and goes through childbirth, a detail overlooked by those who

> compare maternity contracts to sperm donation. ("The Strange Case" 686)

Pollitt adds that the proper corollary to sperm donation is egg donation, a connection that Raymond would probably argue with considering the ease with which men can supply sperm.

To illustrate how confusing the definition of motherhood has become, Pollitt compares the courts' decisions in the Baby M case with a subsequent case filed by Anna Johnson, a woman who acted as a gestational surrogate. In the Whitehead case, Stern's wife was originally deemed to be the proper legal mother of the child, in spite of her lack of a genetic link. In the Johnson case, motherhood was determined by the genetic link Crispina Calvert provided with her egg. Pollitt concludes that "[t]o the small and curious class of English words that have double and contradictory meanings—'moot,' for example, and 'cleave'—the word 'mother' can now be added" ("When is a Mother" 825). Another author who takes issue with the demotion of the role of motherhood is printed in the conservative *National Review*. Maggie Gallagher uses dry wit to make her case and her argument is a bit more graphic: "I hate to be the one to have to point this out, but masturbating into a little cup is not at all like having a baby" (28).

Phyllis Chesler, visiting professor of psychology and women's studies at Brandeis, argues in *Ms*. that the Baby M case exemplifies our society's already skewed valuation of fatherhood and motherhood. "How can this case have happened? Very easily—in a culture that overvalues men, fathers, and money and undervalues women, mothers, and mother-child bonding" (38). For her the Sterns' role in the creation of Baby M is amplified by its equation with "enlightened progress" while Mary Beth Whitehead's role is belittled by its portrayal as "primitive instinct" (39). Chesler explains that Whitehead's claim to the baby had to be devalued so that William Stern's could be acknowledged. "[I]n order for the *idea* of fatherhood to triumph over the *fact* of motherhood, we had to see Bill as the 'birthfather' and Mary Beth as only the surrogate uterus" (39).

Another myth nurtured in the pages of the women's magazine is that reproductive technologies are available to and provided for anyone. In fact, the expense of these services narrows the market to the well off. In 1987, the Sterns paid $25,000 for Baby M (Pollitt "The Strange Case" 684). IVF babies cost anywhere from $67,000 to $800,000

(Neumann et al. 241-242). Most clinics screen potential customers to ensure that they fit their criteria for parenthood (Thom 71). This screening means that single and homosexual men and women can easily be excluded.

The commentators associated with the religiously oriented journals agree with this practice of screening. Sidney Callahan, associate professor of psychology at Mercy College, Dobbs Ferry, New York, writing for the lay Catholic audience of *Commonweal*, explains her carefully qualified approval of reproductive technologies:

> It is ethically appropriate to use alternative reproductive technologies if, and only if, such technologies are making it possible for a normal, socially adequate, heterosexual married couple to have a child as they would, or could, if their infertility were not an obstacle. (Callahan 235)

Callahan's endorsement, while straying from the Church's blanket rejection of artificial reproduction, shows that her position reflects that of the Church on the sanctity of the marital bond. Theologian Jack Moore takes a similar stand in the more ecumenical *Christian Century* by defining a very limited arena in which IVF can be justified: "married couples . . . using their own egg and sperm" (444).

Feminist critics claim that the enhancement-of-motherhood myth has an even greater "phallacy." Phyllis Chesler's critique points out that reproductive procedures are not really provided for wealthy, heterosexual women. They are instead technologies created for wealthy, heterosexual men who, like William Stern, feel "an enormous sense of genetic entitlement" (39). She is not alone in this opinion. Katha Pollitt, Janice Raymond, and Mary Kay Blakely direct the same criticism at the practice of contractual motherhood. Pollitt's is perhaps the most biting:

> But take away the mothers' delusion that they are making babies for other women, and what you have left is what, in cold, hard fact, we already have: the limited-use purchase of women's bodies by men—reproductive prostitution. ("The Strange Case" 684)

The feminists have an even dimmer view of the consequences for the woman who plays the role of contract mother. Mary Thom, senior editor of *Ms.*, argues that the term surrogate minimizes the relationship between the woman and the child she carries, thus diminishing the woman's contribution: "A surrogate mother, pregnant with a fetus that developed from her own *or* another woman's egg is hardly a surrogate anything but is certainly a mother even if not the only mother" (74). Speaking of Mary Beth Whitehead, who did "donate" her own egg, Katha Pollitt explains that using the term surrogate allowed Whitehead's role to be minimized. She was simply the "trivial physical means by which their [the Sterns'] desire . . . was fulfilled" ("The Strange Case" 683). Pollitt believes that Judge Sorkow's decision in the Whitehead case legalized what she defines as reproductive prostitution.

To make a similar point, and mindful of the emotional effect that such a scene will have on her reader, Gallagher describes the "snatching" of the four-month-old Baby M from her crib in Whitehead's home. She adds that at a subsequent visit "Baby M, smelling her mother's milk, nuzzled at Mary Beth's neck, but the court appointed chaperon wouldn't let Baby M nurse" (27). She warns that legal decisions like Sorkow's will create a society in which "judges ponder whether a loving mother may nurse her baby, and where the state can declare a woman *mater non grata*—because someone else outbids her for her child" (30). Like Pollitt, Gallagher likens surrogacy to prostitution, but true to the spirited manner of her discussion, she adds indentured servitude into the equation (30).

The women's magazine depiction of the woman who acts as surrogate mother is that of an altruistic woman who likes being pregnant. She agrees to bear the child because it gives her pleasure and she remains emotionally detached from the child for the best of reasons—so that another woman who craves it can experience motherhood. The feminist commentators disagree with this view of the contractual mother because they believe the practice of surrogacy is a means of exploiting women, especially poor women. They worry that women will be coerced into participating by what seems like a large sum of money. (Katha Pollitt works the price Whitehead was paid—$10,000—out to about $1.50 per hour for the entire pregnancy) ("When is a Mother" 844). Gallagher reports that William Handel, a surrogacy broker, tells the women who work for him that if they try to keep the child "we'll sue you for intentional infliction of emotional distress. You'll have ruined this couple's life. And we'll make it awfully expensive for you to hold on to the child" (30). Certainly none of the "saintly" mothers depicted in the women's magazine reported this kind of treatment.

The feminist commentators argue that contract motherhood invites race and class exploitation. Citing the Anna Johnson custody suit as an example, Pollitt argues that no judge would honor a black woman's claim to a white baby—especially a working-class black woman ("When is a Mother" 842). In her article for *Ms.*, novelist and freelance writer Mary Gordon raises the specter of the baby farm where poor women are used to breed for the rich (26). Finally, Blakely, a women's studies professor and freelance author also writing for *Ms.*, suggests that women drafted into service as contract mothers may some day be classified and paid according to looks and intelligence. With a bitter yet humorous snipe she explains that couples could then choose between the "Saks Fifth Avenue price tag" and the "K-Mart price tag"(20).

These writers extend the exploitation issue to the children who are involved in contract motherhood deals, those watching as a sibling is gestated and handed over to the contracting parents. Callahan's assessment of the emotional detachment required to gestate a child for someone else is damning:

> From another perspective, the woman could also be seen as deliberately producing and selling her baby. What will these practices do to the other children a surrogate may have, or for that matter to other children in the culture? Can children comprehend the fact that mothers make babies and sell them for money? The great primordial reality of interdependency and mutual bonding represented by mother and child is attacked. (239)

Pollitt also couches her objections in terms of the contracting mother's other children: "[H]ow can it not damage a child to watch Mom cheerfully produce and sell its half-sibling while Dad stands idly by?" ("The Strange Case" 688).

An alternate view about the detachment a woman must cultivate to gestate a child for someone else is presented by Malcolm Gladwell and Rochelle Sharpe in *The New Republic*. The authors are both journalists: Gladwell is a contributor to *Insight* magazine, and Sharpe is a reporter for the Washington Bureau of the Gannett News Service. They support the practice of surrogacy if it is managed by a scrupulous broker, one who would provide counseling for women like Mary Beth Whitehead.

Such counseling, they maintain, would have "helped Whitehead *overcome* her bonding with Baby M" (emphasis added 16). Pollitt's rebuttal to this argument is that counseling is just another form of coercion: "True therapy seeks to increase a person's sense of self, not reconcile one to being treated as an instrument" ("The Strange Case" 688).

The female commentators have so far clustered around the women's issues, and especially those involved in contractual motherhood: the degradation of motherhood and the commodification of women's bodies. Their male counterparts cluster around the moral and legal aspects of reproductive technologies, some condemning them just as strongly on moral grounds, others approving such medical services because they allow wanted life to be created.

Professor of ethics at Loyola University in New Orleans, James Gaffney, writing for *Commonweal*, explores the Biblical precedents for surrogacy that many of the other commentators allude to in their discussions. These are precedents his Catholic readership may be curious about since the Church has forbidden any use of modern reproductive technologies. He likens the Mary Beth Whitehead-Baby M case to that of Hagar and Ishmael, reminding the reader that Hagar was punished for challenging Sarai's claim to motherhood, and thereby overstepping the boundaries of her role as substitute mother (240). Gaffney then characterizes the male-heir competition carried out between Rachel and Leah—through their handmaids—as a feminine power struggle. Clearly, he interprets the Biblical precedents as arrangements between women. The feminist commentators would be quick to point out the motivations Rachel and Leah may have had for finding solutions to their infertility: their need to solidify their status by providing their husband with male heirs. (Both were married to Jacob.) Without stating his position overtly, Gaffney discredits contract motherhood by drawing a parallel between modern practice and what appears to be a petty competition between Rachel and Leah. He makes this position clear when he ends his discussion with a question: "Does our own society's disposal of surrogate motherhood as one more commercial transaction, . . . really represent a much higher order of social and moral wisdom than was attained so many centuries ago . . . ?" (242).

Michael Novak, the George Frederick Jewett Chair of Religion and Public Policy at the American Enterprise Institute in Washington, D.C., and columnist John Garvey, both writing for *Commonweal*, view the Baby M case as a problem in legally controlled morality. Novak, who sees the situation as a case of "trafficking in human life" (406), finds the practice to be morally repugnant: "To separate Mrs. Whitehead's *uterus* from her *self* merely by verbal agility is an outrage" (406). Garvey also argues that contractual parenthood is tantamount to slavery. With an understandable Catholic revulsion at the abortion clause in the Baby M contract (the Sterns did not want a child with birth defects), Garvey rejects such legal manipulation of human dignity: "[B]ecause of what it says about our attitudes towards women, children, and humanity in general, surrogacy should be repudiated" (232).

The editors of *Commonweal* also object to contractual motherhood on moral grounds. Presented in a series of editorials printed in reaction to the Baby M case, their objections reflect the position of the Roman Catholic Church on reproductive technologies in general. The editors believe that the practice of contracting for babies is made possible due to a "breakdown in moral understanding," one which fails to recognize that the relationship between reproduction and marital and family bonds should not be severed ("Surrogate-gate" 35). They found the Baby M case appalling, thought that commercial surrogacy should be outlawed ("Birth-Marketing" 692), and believed the New Jersey Supreme court's restoration of Mary Beth Whitehead's parental rights was appropriate ("There Ought" 100). The editors also concluded that the New Jersey decision would be a definitive one, likely to "put an end to the growth of the surrogate-motherhood business. . . " (100). This assessment, made in 1988, failed to take into account the free-market forces that would keep other states from regulating a service that promised to become a lucrative business. The 1988 editorial was the last on the subject for *Commonweal*.

In a *Christian Century* editorial, James M. Wall, Methodist minister and editor of the journal, also poses the Baby M case as a moral question: "Is there anything wrong with allowing individuals to contract to be surrogate mothers?" (99). His answer, that we should not necessarily have access to technologies just because they are possible, takes a swing at science, which he characterizes as a "mindless giant" (99). This is the same mindless giant that is characterized as the miraculous scientific tool of God in the women's magazine. The heartwarming stories narrated there proclaimed God's support for the technological innovations that made mothers' dreams come true. In those tales, God and science seemed to be working together to create miracle babies. Religious commentators like Wall, however, do not share this unconditional support for scientific innovation. Nor do they assume that religious approval should be granted to technology simply because it has the power to give some people what they desire.

Novak views technology as a challenge requiring humanity to establish moral limits: "[N]ew scientific knowledge and technical skills offer so many possibilities that, more and more, the impulse to establish the limits that define who we are. . . is becoming a self-conscious imperative" (407). Callahan, who approves of some reproductive technologies, contends that we should avoid the urge to follow what she calls the "technological imperative" (233). She believes that we cannot allow a combination of human desires and what is technologically possible to decide for us what the right or good course of action may be (233).

In an article published in *America* in 1978, just after the birth of Louise Joy Brown, pioneering medical ethicist and founder of the Kennedy Institute of Ethics at Georgetown University, Andre Hellegers, and Rose E. Kennedy Professor of Christian Ethics at Georgetown, Father Richard McCormick, explore papal proclamations on artificial reproduction. They are looking for any sort of justification for in vitro technology by attempting to determine whether the papal disapproval of the practice was based on its experimental nature or the manner in which it separates the "unitive and procreative dimensions of marital intimacy" (75). Though they find some value in a procedure that allows married people to obey the mandate to reproduce, ultimately they cannot condone in vitro because they "believe that the procedure must be seen in broader social and cultural terms and that, when it is, it is not without serious moral problems" (78). They characterize reproductive technologies as a package deal. If we accept some portion of the practices, then we must also accept practices they enable for the future. In what was a prophetic prediction for 1978, they pose the potential uses to which in vitro could be put:

> And, in time, the next step may well be the surrogate or host womb, where a woman, from medical necessity or convenience, cannot or will not bear her own child. The embryo transfer and child will be carried by a third party. This may seem incredible, but today's

> incredibles are often tomorrow's facts, and it is the part of wisdom to recognize this. (77)

In keeping with the Roman Catholic Church's disapproval of interfering with the "natural" functions of procreation, even the possibility of contractual motherhood is enough to make these two Catholic ethicists find the entire package morally unacceptable.

In contrast to the Roman Catholic's unequivocal stance against reproductive technologies, Jack W. Moore, professor emeritus of religion and philosophy at North Carolina Wesleyan College, Rocky Mount, asks: "Are we not on holy ground where we have no right of passage when we create human beings in a test tube?" (442). His answer, published in the more moderate journal *Christian Century*, is that "[w]e not only have the right but the responsibility to further procreation when it is impaired" (445). Rather than viewing scientific innovation as a disruption of God's natural plan, Moore believes it illustrates how God and man operate as co-workers to improve the "patterns and processes in nature" (445).

Also writing for *Christian Century*, adjunct professor of religion at Roanoke College, Salem, Virginia, Janet Dickey McDowell argues against the Catholic Church's rejection of in vitro on the grounds that the Church's position is inconsistent with its acceptance of other medical technologies (936). She likens IVF to using a dialysis machine in that both mimic normal physiological functions. She believes that "[c]onceptions via IVF ought not simply to be tolerated; they should be celebrated, . . . " (937). Her approval, however, does not extend beyond using IVF for a "loving couple" (937). She does not define who qualifies as a loving couple, but it seems apparent that she refers to married, heterosexual couples. Like many of her colleagues, she does not condone the use of other aspects of reproductive technology.

For a secular opinion of the role that religious morality should play in determining the acceptability of reproductive technology, we can look to Charles Krauthammer, whose article appears in *The New Republic*. Characterized by Maggie Gallagher as *The New Republic*'s "foreign-policy guru. . . [making] a little foray into social issues" (28), Krauthammer's discussion is actually the most substantial of the five articles printed on the topic in the journal. Krauthammer praises the Vatican's Congregation for the Doctrine of the Faith's document on artificial reproduction as "a radical act of resistance to the technological hubris of modern reproductive medicine and to the Frankenstein world that it is rapidly making possible" (17). However, the pragmatic Krauthammer dilutes this praise by ultimately finding the Catholic document to be unrealistic and therefore of little use. Instead he calls the Vatican's rejection of artificial insemination a poor attempt to influence civil law. He proposes that by accomplishing a sort of "moral calculus" we will find our best weapon against reproductive nightmares in "nuance" (21). Thus, Krauthammer joins his more moderate Protestant counterparts in finding that some reproductive practices should be accepted.

After a lull in coverage, the cloning of Dolly the lamb stimulated a more recent discussion in the commentary magazines, possibly because the idea of cloning a human being had seemed part of the realm of science fiction rather than fact. Four of the eight journals have articles—two are news items; two are editorials, and two are critical essays. None endorses the cloning of human beings. Kevin T. Fitzgerald, S.J., writing for *America*, concludes that "social and psychological problems cannot and should not be reduced to genetic or biological solutions" (3). Stephen G. Post's article in *America* presents seven criticisms of cloning. Three of the more compelling are that cloning would eliminate the genetic diversity that is crucial to human survival, encourage organ harvesting, and render men obsolete: "removing male impregnators from the procreative dyad would simply drive the nail into the coffin of fatherhood" (20). His final argument is scriptural. Based on Genesis, Post determines that cloning, like other cultural forces, poses a threat to the core nucleus of family as mandated by Jesus: "Therefore what God has joined together, let no man separate" (21). In a forceful discussion printed in *The Nation*, law professor Patricia J. Williams, examines the possibilities opened up by cloning:

> Imagine what the fashion industry could do with a clone with the right bone structure. Like Barbie, you could style humanity so that all the outfits finally fit. Mozart? Give his DNA a few more codas. Bill Gates and Donald Trump? There'll be lots of them. And we'll need to clone more lawyers in a world where compatible organs can be "farmed." Will questions of "harvest rights" be matters of custodial or property presumption in the new litigation of micro-territorial

imperative? I paid for that kid, it's my DNA, hand over that kidney now. (8).

The last feature of the mythical representation of reproductive technologies presented by the women's magazine is the "GIFT" baby who represents every woman's dream. Naturally, the babies discussed in the pages of the commentary magazine are a bit more problematic; and they present these problems even before the first diaper change. The commentators take up two main issues created by reproductive services. First, children created through contractual motherhood become commodities that can be bought and sold. Second, because in vitro technologies create not only nascent life, but a host of things that can be done with it and to it, the rights and status of these potent little cell groups is debated.

The women's magazines focus on the baby as the cherished goal who makes all the suffering worthwhile. Naturally, it is assumed, these babies will be loved all the more because they were wanted so terribly. But is it possible for a baby to be wanted too much? Many of the commentators believe that the extensive measures to which some would-be parents will go are by their nature harmful to the child produced, bought and sold. Instead of entering the world as someone's responsibility, these children are responsible for the happiness of those who fought so hard to create them. Regardless of which interests they represent—sacred, secular, liberal, or conservative—the commentators agree that being bought and sold is not healthy for the child at the heart of the transaction. "Do we sense . . . some lingering suspicion that baby deals are not quite like pork belly deals? Oh well, give it time" ("Infantrepreneurs" 228). Is contractual motherhood the equivalent of trading pork bellies? The comparison seems rather harsh and since this remark was printed in a *Commonweal* editorial, one could attribute it to a Catholic sensitivity to the potential commodification of life inherent in contractual motherhood. The editors of *Commonweal* are not alone, however, in their condemnation of a practice that they feel makes commodities out of children, or in their pork belly comparison for that matter. Secular critic Katha Pollitt makes a similar quip in reference to the Baby M case: "You'd think she had signed a contract to trade sow bellies at $5 . . . " (685).

Commentators who are not caught up in being vitriolic about the practice explain their objections to producing children via contract motherhood a bit more rationally. Representing the Catholic community, Sidney Callahan explains her disapproval in religious terms: "When one is *begotten not made*, then one shares equally with one's parents in the ongoing transmission of the gift of life. . ." (emphasis added 237). Since Callahan approves of the limited use of in vitro for married couples, her objection is to the introduction into the marital relationship of third party genes. This introduction constitutes the deliberate manipulation of life—she calls it "drafting"—to which she objects.

In her critique of contract motherhood, Blakely focuses on the expectations that contract parents would inevitably have for a purchased child: "Even a surrogate baby, carefully gened and legally guaranteed, cannot live up to such fantastic expectations" (20). Writing for the moderate *Christian Century*, Linda Delloff, from the POLIS Research Center at Indiana University-Purdue University, is also concerned about parental expectations, though in a slightly different context. Her piece is a response to the birth of the first baby born from donated Nobel prize-winning sperm. She believes such parents would compromise the quality of their offsprings' lives regardless of the outcome of their genetic experiment: "[p]ity such babies whose lives are planned for them before they emerge from the womb" (749). She also believes they have wandered into God's territory. "When Christ commanded, 'Suffer little children to come unto me, . . . ' he wasn't just referring to those with IQs of 130" (750). Maggie Gallagher's piece sums up the problem of responsibility nicely: "The child cannot obligate her [the contract mother], she obligates it: It is a product, conceived for sale and use" (30).

The second of the two impediments to the "happy ending" of the women's magazine fairy tale is one which excites a great deal of moral and ethical debate. The religious critics, already deeply concerned with the question of when life begins, shudder at the thought of petri dishes full of disposable embryos. It makes perfect sense that the Catholic team Hellegers and McCormick reject in vitro in part because of "the disturbing question of zygote loss" (76). They add a concern for potential birth defects that could result from the procedures: "Here we have an experimental procedure undertaken to benefit prospective parents with the risks being borne by the child and without its consent or any possibility of consent" (76).

The second of the two articles printed in *America* examines a legal decision that also happens to support Catholic tenets about the definition of life. The author, Joseph Allegretti, is a professor of law and assistant director for law and religious ethics at the Center for Health Policy and Ethics at Creighton University in Omaha, Nebraska. Allegretti addresses one of the more interesting cases caused by in vitro practices. In a 1989 divorce suit, custody of seven frozen embryos was awarded to the wife based on the judge's decision that they were human beings. Though the custody decision was overturned after Allegretti's article was published, his discussion of the law involved in the case is very reasonable and persuasive. He explains that the judge had to choose between classifying the embryos as property or children. Allegretti recognizes that embryos are not children, but he makes his case that they are "more like children than they are like a chair" (305). He never invokes theology in this discussion, basing his reasoning entirely on the legal dilemma.

The editors of *Commonweal* address the problem of aborting nascent life in an editorial that was published immediately after the birth of Louise Joy Brown. They acknowledge that ending the life of a fertilized egg may not be considered abortion by some, but very practically point out that "there is little reason to think that the manufacturing principles of quality control can halt there" since Leslie Brown agreed in writing that she would abort a defective fetus ("Test-Tube Babies" 548). *Christian Century* editor and David Rice Professor of Ethics at Rice University, James Sellers, also responds to Louise Brown's birth by pointing out the moral problems inherent in in vitro. Remarking on how "placid" the discussion of test-tube technology has been, Sellers reminds the reader that in vitro invites the same question being argued in the debate over abortion: when human life begins. He takes an incremental position on the problem, arguing that the embryo does not have full rights at conception, "but it begins to accumulate rights as it develops toward humanness" (757). Based on Sellers' 1978 position, some interesting legal problems could now be posed in response to the latest technologies: determining at just what stage its human rights would be frozen when an embryo is preserved for banking, deciding which embryos have the right to live when a couple elects to undergo selective abortion (the oldest?), or establishing which cloned embryo preceded the others in the procedure.

Janet McDowell, writing in 1983, takes a position that illustrates how quickly our technological capabilities surpass our moral proclamations. Her approval of IVF procedures is based on the clinics' practice of implanting all embryos created. If clinics were to retain embryos, she argues, this practice would come under a different moral heading and would not reflect on the acceptability of IVF itself (937). It is interesting to note how far McDowell's position is from the Roman Catholic's "package deal" view of reproductive technologies. One wonders what her reaction was to Britain's recent embryo-cleansing: all frozen embryos that had been stored more than five years and that were not claimed by "parents" were thawed and disposed of.

Another religious commentator does regard reproductive advances as an all-or-nothing proposition. A Lutheran pastor, Richard Neuhaus is also the director of New York's Rockford Institute Center on Religion and Society. The author of *Commentary*'s sole discussion of reproductive technologies, Neuhaus views them as a vehicle for a new eugenics. His objection is not to the technological advances themselves, but to the practices they enable. For him the "real growth areas in the synthetic-child business" (16) include genetic engineering and fetal experimentation. Acknowledging that the creation of life in the laboratory also allows for the destruction of life in the laboratory, Neuhaus explains that he is far more concerned that our technological capabilities will allow us to create a socially engineered society (17). To illustrate how offended he is by the experimental use of fetal tissue, he presents a morally repugnant example. A California woman proposed that she be artificially inseminated with her father's sperm so she could abort the subsequent fetus and have it used in an attempt to cure the father's Alzheimer's disease (18). In a society that has no clear moral guidelines for such medical possibilities, Neuhaus speculates sardonically that her "act of love . . . would no doubt meet with overwhelming support on the Phil Donahue show . . ."(18).

Religious debate about the status of embryonic life is not necessarily unique to the religious journals. Former Jesuit priest Malachi Martin's condemnation of in vitro technology in the *National Review* contains more references to Christian morality than do many of those written for the strictly religious journals. In "Test-Tube Morality," Martin rails at a society which easily accepts a whole menu of scientific innovations that Aquinas and Augustine could never have foreseen, and which sets policies while consciously excluding "all considerations of a religious nature" (1285). Martin considers the destruction of embryonic life to be "multiple infanticide" (1285). He shudders on the page at the morals that allow some "non-Christians" to endorse or engage in actions that create an atmosphere of "[e]very embryo for itself, and the trash-can take the hindmost!" (1285). He expresses his moral horror over fetal experimentation by making use of language that is both graphic and vitriolic: Non-Christians endorse the use of a drug that "permits the abortion of the fetus alive and ready to have its head cut off and its body cut up by the medical researchers" (1285). Apparently he believes that his own charged language is necessary compensation for the use of what he calls "Easyspeak": euphemisms like "pregnancy termination" that make certain technological practices more palatable (1285).

For a secular view that rejects both religious and feminist concerns about reproductive technologies, we can turn to *The New Republic* and William Tucker's version of "In Vitro Veritas." Tucker, a contributing editor of *Harper's*, counters concerns about embryos being "'flushed down the toilet,'" (out of the bottle into the bowl?) by explaining that "human females produce eggs at a rate of one per month" (15). He believes that the in vitro procedures will never involve more than one embryo implantation at a time. This article was printed in 1981, before it became common practice to implant multiple embryos into women undergoing in vitro procedures. It seems unlikely though that even with this new twist Tucker would relax his endorsement of in vitro because he views any argument over its value as a cover for the anti-abortion movement's agenda. "The gaggle of opposition to *in vitro* fertilization has one thing in common: religious fundamentalism, whether sacred or secular" (16). Tucker's "gaggle" is made up of several groups, all of whom he considers to be extremists: they include a "robust cross-fertilization between right-to-lifers and some of the anti-technological extremists on the fringes of the environmental movement," and "some of the radical factions of the women's movement" (16). Whatever its composition, it is clear that to Tucker the noisy opposition to in vitro should be considered just as seriously as one would a swarming flock of geese.

In his version of "In Vitro Veritas," Robert Bazell, the science correspondent for NBC News, addresses the problem of selective abortion that was raised by the birth of quintuplets in 1988. Though these particular quintuplets survived and were healthy, their birth made public the dilemma posed by the multiple pregnancies that current in vitro practices often create. Bazell calls for an end to the secrecy that surrounds what the medical profession calls "'embryo reduction procedure'" (12). To illustrate the problem, Bazell quotes Dr. David Navot, an IVF expert: "It's like hearsay. . . . People who are dealing with IVF and occasionally get into multiple pregnancies know where to go. But there are no statistics, no numbers'" (12). Pregnancy reduction is not a moral problem for Bazell, however, instead he is concerned that we set public policy. He explains that he understands the secrecy. The doctors are saving one or two fetuses and possibly the mother by terminating the others. "People whose main work is helping couples have babies certainly do not want anti-abortion demonstrators at their door" (12). Because the future holds the possibility of new procedures such as cloning and what is now known as gestational surrogacy, Bazell wants a public discussion. He believes that we should decide as a society which of these technologies we want to use and which we do not before "someone gets enough signatures on a petition to put a stop to all of it" (13). For Bazell, the danger seems to be not that technology will inappropriately legislate morality, but that morality will inappropriately legislate technology. I would like to lock him in a room with Malachi Martin and see who emerges with a moral black eye.

On November 19, 1997, Bobby McCaughey, a small town Iowa woman, gave birth to the world's first surviving septuplets. Multiple births are more and more common these days and most triplet and quadruplet births barely make the news, but septuplets were enough to make the whole nation take notice. John Garvey's discussion of the birth in *Commonweal* addresses the same issues that Bazell worried over in 1988, but Garvey contends that the choices presented by multiple pregnancies cheapen life (7). "But babies are not products. There is something terrifying about the fact that babies are aborted for being the wrong sex (usually female) and something chilling in the 'lifeboat' scenario of 'selective reduction,' where some lives are tossed out to save others" (7). Though he praises the McCaugheys for deciding against selective reduction, he does not believe that gestating seven babies is the ideal choice either. Our desire to be so in control over our lives (by creating children when it is not naturally possible) is the problem, Garvey says, of living in a secular and Godless society.

By responding mainly to the cases that Linda Gordon characterizes as "arrangements gone wrong," those who debate reproductive technologies in the commentary journals often miss the opportunity to examine some of the practices that go unquestioned in the courts. The "happy endings" that populate the fantasy case histories in the women's magazines offer some interesting moral and ethical dilemmas that have not been addressed here. Some examples from the cases presented in chapter three include: the posthumous creation of children who will never know one genetic parent; the use of IVF and AI to create children for parents with serious medical conditions; children created out of wedlock by single parents; and the technologically incestuous practice of a grandmother carrying fetuses for her daughter. If the writers of the commentary journals would pick up one of the women's magazines from time to time, they would find some very good fuel for their discussion. Still, the discussion we have examined here attacks the women's magazine fantasy on all levels. If the reader of the women's magazine were to pick up a commentary journal from time to time, she would find it impossible to read her next issue of *Good Housekeeping* through the same eyes.

NOTES

1. Raymond's figures represent "traditional" IVF procedures. At least one clinic using the newest GIFT and ZIFT procedures under optimal conditions reports success rates as high as 40-50 percent (Elmer-Dewitt "Making Babies" 61). Still, the norm is probably much lower than this.

2. Since the female reproductive system shuts down when all of its egg follicles have produced eggs, superovulation undoubtedly means that women who go through these procedures will experience menopause earlier than they would otherwise. Earlier onset of menopause will mean that the hormonal levels will be changed earlier, increasing the risk of breast cancer. Some women will use estrogen replacement therapy (ERT) to counteract this possibility, but ERT poses alternative risks—endometrial cancer (Seaman and Seaman 331). While these risks may be acceptable to the woman who has fertility problems and weighs them next to her desire to have a child, the otherwise healthy woman who "volunteers" to donate eggs will experience the same risks.

CHAPTER FIVE

Gynecology at the Breakfast Table

Ben Bradlee, managing editor of *The Washington Post*, is credited with saying that the "news is the first rough draft of history" (Andrews 632). Indeed, our news publications have many of the qualities of a rough draft. Because of time constraints, news texts are rarely as penetrating as those in the commentary journal. Rather than representing one consistent point of view, the news reporter compiles a story out of the facts, testimonials, and diverse opinions he or she gathers together on the topic in question. Depending on his or her level of expertise and impartiality, the reporter will be more or less capable of orchestrating the disparate voices called together in the article. This group agent differs from the diverse agents of the commentary journal in that the commentators, while representing a variety of opinions, remain consistent within their particular ideologies and discourse communities. The news writer, however, brings together and tries to manage the representatives of many different discourse communities. The result is often more like a cacophony of voices than an organized debate. Because of this blend of voices, the gynecological case history that appears in the news media offers the elements of the fairy tale alongside the critical debate of the commentator.

The news writer's purpose also differs from that of the commentator or the author of the women's magazine piece. The reporter attempts to act as an impartial informant, notifying the reader of important events, dangerous practices, and unethical behaviors. The assumption that the news can be reported impartially means that the press is awarded a great deal of credibility, and it is considered by many readers to be highly objective.

The readership of the news media is quite varied. This large group can easily include the audiences of both the women's magazine and the commentary journal, though those who read both will award them different positions in the home. The women's magazine will probably go from the check-out stand to the nightstand, while the commentary journal will remain proudly displayed on the coffee table. The news media may travel about the house a bit more, but for this chapter I have located them at the breakfast table because one of the first places one finds the newspaper is folded neatly beside the morning toast and coffee. The news magazine may or may not be found there as well, but locating gynecology at the breakfast table will provoke fewer blushes than locating it at the commode.[1]

The nation's two most popular news magazines are *Time* and *Newsweek*. These two magazines have been in publication for most of the twentieth century; *Time* was founded in 1923 and *Newsweek* in 1933. They have circulations of 4.5 million and 3 million respectively (Katz and Katz 819, 821). Together they cannot even challenge the total readership of the women's service magazines, but they do account for a much larger audience than the commentary journal. Often running the same headlines each week, these two news magazines are remarkably similar. Katz and Katz describe *Time*'s viewpoint as that of the "conservative, middle-of-the-road American" (821). They distinguish *Newsweek*'s approach from *Time*'s by defining it as more liberal and socially conscious, characterizing its target reader as more affluent, compassionate, and endowed with an intellectual appreciation (819). Published weekly, these two periodicals are responsible for 87—nearly half—of the news magazines' 166 articles covering reproductive technology between 1977 and 1997. *Time* printed 45 articles and *Newsweek* printed 42 articles.

A sampling of the daily news media's coverage of reproductive technology will be taken from the *New York Times*, founded in 1851 and with a paid circulation of 1.2 million (Ulrich's 54), the *Los Angeles Times*, founded in 1881 and with a paid circulation of 1.1 million (7), and the *Houston Chronicle*, founded in 1901 and with a paid circulation of 419,759 (79). The East Coast's *New York Times* is the authoritative newspaper, considered to "set the standard by which all other newspapers are measured" (Katz and Katz 825). On the West Coast, the *Los Angeles Times*, by virtue of its location in California, the "surrogate state," has the advantage of being on the spot for many of the breaking

CHAPTER FIVE

Gynecology at the Breakfast Table

Ben Bradlee, managing editor of *The Washington Post*, is credited with saying that the "news is the first rough draft of history" (Andrews 632). Indeed, our news publications have many of the qualities of a rough draft. Because of time constraints, news texts are rarely as penetrating as those in the commentary journal. Rather than representing one consistent point of view, the news reporter compiles a story out of the facts, testimonials, and diverse opinions he or she gathers together on the topic in question. Depending on his or her level of expertise and impartiality, the reporter will be more or less capable of orchestrating the disparate voices called together in the article. This group agent differs from the diverse agents of the commentary journal in that the commentators, while representing a variety of opinions, remain consistent within their particular ideologies and discourse communities. The news writer, however, brings together and tries to manage the representatives of many different discourse communities. The result is often more like a cacophony of voices than an organized debate. Because of this blend of voices, the gynecological case history that appears in the news media offers the elements of the fairy tale alongside the critical debate of the commentator.

The news writer's purpose also differs from that of the commentator or the author of the women's magazine piece. The reporter attempts to act as an impartial informant, notifying the reader of important events, dangerous practices, and unethical behaviors. The assumption that the news can be reported impartially means that the press is awarded a great deal of credibility, and it is considered by many readers to be highly objective.

The readership of the news media is quite varied. This large group can easily include the audiences of both the women's magazine and the commentary journal, though those who read both will award them different positions in the home. The women's magazine will probably go from the check-out stand to the nightstand, while the commentary journal will remain proudly displayed on the coffee table. The news media may travel about the house a bit more, but for this chapter I have located them at the breakfast table because one of the first places one finds the newspaper is folded neatly beside the morning toast and coffee. The news magazine may or may not be found there as well, but locating gynecology at the breakfast table will provoke fewer blushes than locating it at the commode.[1]

The nation's two most popular news magazines are *Time* and *Newsweek*. These two magazines have been in publication for most of the twentieth century; *Time* was founded in 1923 and *Newsweek* in 1933. They have circulations of 4.5 million and 3 million respectively (Katz and Katz 819, 821). Together they cannot even challenge the total readership of the women's service magazines, but they do account for a much larger audience than the commentary journal. Often running the same headlines each week, these two news magazines are remarkably similar. Katz and Katz describe *Time*'s viewpoint as that of the "conservative, middle-of-the-road American" (821). They distinguish *Newsweek*'s approach from *Time*'s by defining it as more liberal and socially conscious, characterizing its target reader as more affluent, compassionate, and endowed with an intellectual appreciation (819). Published weekly, these two periodicals are responsible for 87—nearly half—of the news magazines' 166 articles covering reproductive technology between 1977 and 1997. *Time* printed 45 articles and *Newsweek* printed 42 articles.

A sampling of the daily news media's coverage of reproductive technology will be taken from the *New York Times*, founded in 1851 and with a paid circulation of 1.2 million (Ulrich's 54), the *Los Angeles Times*, founded in 1881 and with a paid circulation of 1.1 million (7), and the *Houston Chronicle*, founded in 1901 and with a paid circulation of 419,759 (79). The East Coast's *New York Times* is the authoritative newspaper, considered to "set the standard by which all other newspapers are measured" (Katz and Katz 825). On the West Coast, the *Los Angeles Times*, by virtue of its location in California, the "surrogate state," has the advantage of being on the spot for many of the breaking out in the baby department while on a shopping expedition. In this venue, rather than evoking sympathy, the story reinforces the view created of her as an obsessive woman (70).

While most reporters take great pains to explain all of the technology behind in vitro, they do not report much about the physical pain such procedures cause. One account describes the IVF procedure, including egg removal, with no reference to pain. Then the reporter tells his reader that the embryos are put into a Teflon catheter and inserted into the uterus "usually with no discomfort" (Clark 106). It is odd that the reporter felt it necessary to explain that the implantation procedure is usually pain-free, while omitting any mention of the other more painful practices involved.

A *Time* profile of Arlette Schweitzer, who we will recall carried twins for her daughter, also minimizes the amount of physical pain she endured. Her comments about having to inject herself with fertility drugs for 89 days are colored by her motives: she is a mother making a sacrifice for her daughter's happiness. She explains that while she still has scars on her hips from the hormone injections, "'[f]or 89 days I think you could even walk on coals if you had to'" (qtd. in Nash 58). More recent articles do address the psychological pain experienced by infertile couples, especially when reproductive technologies do not produce the genetically-related children they are seeking. A 1996 *New York Times* series on infertility devotes an entire column to how infertile couples cope with their inability to conceive. "'There's a feeling of being left behind in the life cycle. . . . There're baby showers. Open school day. Christmas. Hanukkah. Things as difficult as being left out at Halloween. My God, you can't play and you want to. You're left out and it hurts'" (Madsen qtd. in Lee 4).

The news media can be counted on for profiles of contract mothers—the nature of their "service" makes for good news stories. Arlette Schweitzer is a perfect example of the totally altruistic woman who is a great mother in her own right. Schweitzer is characterized in *Time* as a "gutsy South Dakota grandma" (Nash 58). She is gutsy because at 42 she became the country's first "gestational surrogate," but more importantly, she did it for her daughter. Calling her a grandma emphasizes her genetic relationship to the twins she carried rather than her biological relationship to them, reminding us that these relationships are now often separate and distinct. The title of grandma also highlights Schweitzer's relationship to her daughter, making it a more important biological tie than the one between her and the two babies she nurtured for nine months.

In a rather roundabout way, Schweitzer is also characterized as saintly: when she speaks her voice is "as clear and as strong as a church bell" (58). Though her actions violate her church's official position on artificial reproduction, Schweitzer's rationale is presented as a logical outcome of her faith: "With refreshing, down-to-earth pragmatism, Arlette, a devout Roman Catholic, says she had no doubts about her decision. 'If medical science affords that opportunity, why not take it?'" (58).

Another case, heralded in the *Houston Chronicle* by the headline "53-year-old gives birth to grandson" marks a similar act of "motherly love." Because her daughter-in-law was unable to bear children, a 53-year-old woman underwent hormone treatments to jump-start her reproductive system and carry her son's child. Though the article quotes a representative from the American Fertility Society as having "serious reservations about any attempt to produce pregnancy beyond the ordinary childbearing age" ("53-year-old" 5A), the story glosses over a powerful potential controversy raised by both this case and the Schweitzer case: the ethical implications of a woman carrying her son's or daughter's child. In a more recent birth, an Italian woman gestated an embryo for her brother after his wife's death. The *New York Time*'s 1995 article does raise the incest issue by quoting neo-Facist Parliament member Alessandra Mussolini, who calls the birth "'immoral and incestuous'" (Tagliabue A8). However, the expert who is probably both more sympathetic and authoritative is Rita Levi Montalcini, the 1986 Nobel Prize recipient for medicine. She characterizes the birth as an "'act of generosity'" (A8). This problem of technological incest has largely been avoided by the media. The use of eggs and sperm from sponsoring parents seems to create a condition of technological purity for the woman who allows her uterus to be used in this fashion. Instead of being considered impure for her actions, the woman who gestates the fetus[es] is actually treated in much the same way as the Virgin Mary was. God is simply acting through her, facilitated by technology.

A *Newsweek* profile of several women who have acted as surrogates makes this same comparison with the virgin birth. When challenged by a fellow church member about the morality of her actions, one woman's retort was that "'Mary was a surrogate for God'"

(Cassem qtd. in Kantrowitz 46). By equating her actions with the virgin birth, the woman is able to retain her purity and piety without question.

Another woman profiled in the *Newsweek* piece exemplifies the altruism attributed to these women. She explains that she became a contract mother because she worked for three fertility doctors and saw the anguish the infertile women experienced (Kantrowitz 46). Finally, a third was so determined to carry someone else's child that she persisted despite a family war with her in-laws. Though they threatened to disown her husband and take her children away, she went ahead with the procedure and became pregnant (48). In the news piece she explains that the experience has made her marriage stronger. For all of these women, the drive to motherhood—albeit contractual—overpowers any obstacles standing in their paths.

Newsweek editor Barbara Kantrowitz, the author of the piece, does acknowledge that women who contract to be mothers do not always do so for the purist of motives. She cites a study that describes three main reasons women become contractual mothers: "money, a desire to be pregnant and an interest in reconciling some past birth-related trauma" (47). After profiling the typical contract mother, the author explains that this portrait matches Mary Beth Whitehead perfectly (47). Apparently, her application for broker Noel Keane made her seem like the ideal woman for the job. Her motives fit easily into the first and second categories above. By describing Whitehead's surrogacy application as "poignantly naive" (47), the author uses the case to call into question the definition of the "perfect surrogate."

Another sympathetic surrogacy profile is presented in the *New York Time*'s 1997 story of Sharon Ogrin, the wife of professional golfer David Ogrin. Ogrin carried a child for her sister, who was infertile: "Jaimie Allynn Gomez . . . is now a happy, healthy, 7-month-old who will spend the holidays crawling beneath the Christmas tree and being thoroughly spoiled by the family" (Brown C1). The article is as much about David Ogrin as it is about his wife, portraying him as completely supportive of the arrangement. He believes that the baby's birth proved to his daughter that prayers come true.

The news media coverage also shows how the relationship between contracting mother and child is downplayed while the relationship with the sponsoring mother is emphasized. One contract mom explains: "'It wasn't my baby. There was no attachment at all. I knew from the beginning that this was their baby, not mine" (qtd. in Kantrowitz 48).

Whitehead's early relationship with Elizabeth Stern is characterized as very close: "'When I first talked to Mary Beth, it was like talking to my sister'" (Stern qtd. in Kantrowitz 48). David Ogrin made name tags for his sister-in-law's baby shower. His wife's read "Oven" and his read "Womb for Rent" (Brown C3). Later in this discussion the Anna Johnson case will demonstrate just how detached gestating can become: a woman who nurtures a child made from someone else's genetic material can be determined to be a "genetic stranger" to that child, and therefore of no consequence once the gestation is complete.

As in the women's magazine, the egg donor is represented in *Newsweek* as simply a new type of surrogate, motivated by the same altruistic feelings as she who "donates" her womb for nine months. "Whether she is helping a desperate sister, friend, colleague, or a stranger, the average donor acts out of altruism" (Ames 60). A donor identified only by a pseudonym—Elizabeth—makes an analogy that shows the characteristic detachment requisite for someone in this occupation: "'I may have given the yeast, but the bread isn't mine'" (61). Another donor who has made eleven egg donations is depicted as a sort of "super-egg mom." She meets with and approves the couples ahead of time. Those who have been successful send annual pictures of the five children that have been born from her eggs. Of her role in helping to create these families she says, "'I get sheer enjoyment out of it'" (61).

A *New York Times* article on egg donation shows both sides of the issue, quoting from medical ethicist Dr. Arthur Caplan: "'If we don't believe in buying and selling babies, then why are we comfortable buying and selling sperm and eggs?" (qtd. in Hoffman 1). For balance, the opinion of a woman who has acted both as a contract mother and an egg donor is also cited: "'I feel like a good soldier.'" She imagines God asking for her service: "'Hey girl, I've done a lot for you and now I want you to do something for Me.'" (Loustalot qtd. in Hoffman 10).

In the women's magazines several women are profiled who sued for custody of the children they created for others. Those that retained the image of the good mother sued for custody for the same sort of altruistic reasons that motivated them to act as contract mothers in the first place. A California case profiled in the *Los Angeles Times* fits this category. In this situation, a woman who was the genetic mother of the child she conceived for a couple sued for custody because the couple split up. The series of articles covering the case begins with an introduction to the three "parents" debating custody.

The sponsoring mother, Cynthia Moschetta, is presented as a victim; she has been left by her husband and now stands to lose the six-month-old daughter she took maternity leave to care for. We can hardly avoid feeling sympathy for her, especially after this quote:

> "He offered me money to leave," Cynthia Moschetta said, breaking into tears. "He would tell me that I don't have any rights, because I'm not the mother. I told him that there was no amount of money in the world that he could give me that would replace Marissa." (Efron "A 3-Way Fight" A32)

After reading this quote, we already have a negative view of Robert Moschetta, the man who told his wife he was moving out and taking the baby with him. In dispute is a document he had the contracting mother, Elvira Jordan, sign giving him sole custody of the child. Jordan's attorneys claimed that she does not read English and she did not read or understand the document. Moschetta's comment about the document is that he was just "wrap[ping] up the paperwork" (A32). This explanation makes him sound like the sort of man who would take advantage of the woman's inability to read English. He appears to be just the type of man the feminist commentators claim this technology was created for. By offering his estranged wife money to leave, he highlights just who was "buying" the child in this case.

On the other hand, Jordan is characterized as a caring mother who, like Patty Nowakowski, has been placed in the position of having to protect her child. According to her attorney, she is "'not a surrogate kicking up trouble'" (Kellogg qtd. in Efron A32). As the genetic mother of the child she "wanted her daughter to be raised by a happy, loving couple" (A3). If the Moschettas had remained married, she would have obediently handed the child over to them. Their separation and ensuing divorce made the usual surrogate-style compliance impossible.

The reporter on this story, Sonni Efron, explains that the judge's decision will affect the definition of parenthood, having "implications for gay parents, stepparents and others who rear children in non-traditional families" (A3). She cites experts in surrogacy arrangements and reproductive law: James Boskey of Seton Hall University Law

School; Nina F. Kellogg, a Los Angeles psychologist and surrogacy broker; Marjorie M. Schultz, a UC Berkeley law professor; and Martha Field, A Harvard Law School professor. Each has a different view of the case and its potential for changing contractual motherhood in California.

A follow-up story by Efron tells the reader about the legal decision: "In a ruling that could bolster the rights of surrogate mothers in California, a Superior Court judge in Orange County ruled Thursday that a surrogate mother is the legal parent of the baby girl she bore for a couple who are now divorcing" ("Surrogate" A30). Legal expert Martha A. Field is quoted registering her surprise that Jordan won the case. She explains that contracting mothers often lack the resources for fighting such battles against more financially stable adoptive couples. The judge's decision in this case is something of a surprise to another legal expert, James Boskey, because ruling the surrogacy contract unenforceable jeopardizes such contracts in the already burgeoning California surrogacy industry (A31). The judge's disapproval of contractual motherhood is unmistakable; she declares invalid any contract that requires "'irreversible pre-conception relinquishment of parental rights without consideration of the best interests of the child'" (Weiben Stock qtd. in Efron A30).

The final article in the news series reports that Jordan has been given joint custody with the child's father. This reporter calls Jordan the "surrogate mother" (Lait "Judge" A3). His use of this term so late in the case is evidence of the strength of the expression. Jordan has already been declared the child's legal mother. She is indeed the child's biological mother; yet she still wears the surrogate label. The reporter also points out that the judge, by giving Jordan joint custody, has gone against the court expert's recommendation. We read Jordan's reaction and then the father's. She "collapsed with emotion," (A3) and he "strongly denounced the ruling" (A27).

The *Los Angeles Times* also printed three discussions of the Jordan case. One reports the critical reaction of family experts to Judge Weiben Stock's decision. James Boskey, the family law professor who is quoted in the previous article, characterizes the decision as unhealthy for the child (Lait "Family" A31). Dr. Stephen Herman, a psychiatrist from Yale, says that joint custody is a panacea that rarely works (A31), and Dr. Justin Call, the head of UC Irvine's Child and Adolescent Psychiatry Department, calls the joint custody arrangement "doomed for failure" (A31). To counter these opinions, the reporter gives us a different kind of expert—Mary Beth Whitehead-Gould. Introduced as the "surrogate mother in the watershed 'Baby M' case," she says "I wish I had gotten joint custody. . . . I think it is the best situation for the child" (A31). Placed next to the authoritative opinions of psychiatrists and lawyers, hers sounds rather self-serving and naive.

The final article on this case is an editorial calling for government regulation of the surrogacy industry. The editor characterizes the outcome of the case as "ultimately disappointing. . . [with] no rights for the sponsoring mother, day-care-provider status for the surrogate, and certain confusion for child and father" ("Tangled" B5). The writer seems to find the "elevated status of a surrogate" most disturbing. Elvira Jordan is referred to as the surrogate, never even the surrogate mother and, according to the author, a surrogate is "a person whose womb was let for rent . . ." (B5). The message of the editorial is that government must regulate this industry—called "this brave new world of surrogacy" in a reference to Alduous Huxley's novel—before more women acting as surrogates are allowed to become "an important longterm player in a child's upbringing" (B5).

If the *Los Angeles Times*' coverage of the Elvira Jordan case shows a somewhat mixed attitude toward her custody suit, the *Time* and *Newsweek* coverage of the Mary Beth Whitehead case is more sympathetic than might be expected for the woman who has come to represent the wicked witch of surrogacy. In a commentary essay in *Time*, senior writer Roger Rosenblatt takes a strong stand against contractual motherhood, using the Baby M case as the focal point of his discussion. His interpretation of the arrangement between Whitehead and Stern is that "she was paid to experience maternal love, the forced cessation of that love, and a whole range of feelings in the process that are not ordinarily put up for sale" (88). Rosenblatt likens the deal struck between Whitehead and Stern to the one that Faust made with the Devil: "In a way, neither Stern nor Whitehead had a claim to the service they were dealing with, any more than Faust had a claim to the soul he dealt the Devil" (88).

In two *Time* news pieces on the case, Richard Lacayo allows a variety of experts to give opinions on the Whitehead case. In the first piece, he quotes Whitehead's anguished cry as she turned her daughter over to the Sterns: "Oh God, what have I done?" ("Whose Child" 56). Lacayo uses the case to pose two contradictory questions: If society allows such arrangements, "[h]as it imperiled its most venerable notions of kinship and the bond between mother and child?" (56), and if the practice is prohibited, "has a promising way for childless couples to have families been denied them?" (56). Instead of answering these questions himself, Lacayo presents an array of expert opinions denouncing the practice of contractual motherhood. The New Jersey Bishops of the Roman Catholic Church believe that the practice "'exploits a child as a commodity and exploits a woman as a babymaker'" (qtd. in Lacayo 58). Rabbi Moses Tendler worries that contract motherhood will allow people to practice a sort of piecemeal slavery, buying the use of specific organs (58). Bioethicist Arthur Caplan does not think people should be gestating babies for money (58). Norman Robbins, family law attorney, says children are not goods or property (58), and Elizabeth Kane, the much publicized "first surrogate" who later changed her mind about the practice, explains that the woman acting as surrogate is not granted any rights (58). In this coverage, the weight of such negative expert opinion denounces the practice.

The *Newsweek* coverage of the Whitehead case is also sympathetic, although author Kantrowitz surrounds her explanation of Whitehead's circumstances with profiles of women who have acted as surrogates without incident. She balances their positive experiences by quoting Elizabeth Kane's most well known line: "'All you're doing is transferring the pain from one woman to another, from a woman who is in pain from her infertility to a woman who has to give up her baby'" (46). An effective means of bringing Whitehead's point of view home to the reader is the description of her emotional reaction to giving the baby up. "But her first night without the baby was agony" (49). Even better is Tuesday Whitehead's account of the day her little sister was snatched sleeping from her crib. Screaming "No," Tuesday chased after the men, an FBI agent and a private investigator, and helplessly tried to stop them by beating one of them on the back with the only weapon she had at hand, her hairbrush (49).

The wicked surrogate "kicking up trouble" who has probably received the worst publicity is Anna Johnson, the woman who acted as a gestational surrogate and then sued for custody of the child. In a *Los Angeles Times Magazine* article she is characterized as manipulative, dishonest, and selfish. She appears to be suing for custody "out of complex motivations that seemed dominated by pure spite toward the better-fixed couple who she believed was neglecting her" (Kasindorf 12).

Johnson's was the first custody case in which the contract mother was not also the genetic mother of the child in dispute. The Calverts had to argue that the genetic material they supplied to create the child in Anna Johnson's womb was indeed their property. Their lawyer is quoted in the *Los Angeles Times* as saying that "'the genetic parents have more right to the baby. . . . Genetics are the property of the parents who provided them'" (Van Deusen qtd. in Gewertz A22). In the Davis case debated in *America* by Joseph Allegretti, just the opposite argument was made; the embryos were determined to be human beings and not property.

A follow-up article tells of the birth of the baby boy and depicts it as a "legal and emotional firestorm" (Gewertz A35). The lawyers are in a "frenzy of activity," "rushing" and "racing" to the hospital to make sure that Johnson does not bring the baby home before custody is determined. In contrast to all of this activity around Johnson, Cris Calvert is depicted as sitting quietly at home, waiting to see if she can visit the baby. She is the meek and submissive mother, just waiting to see if she will be allowed to raise her child. She tells the reporter "'I'm still so shaky, . . . I'm real excited, but I'm also worried. I know in my heart that he's our baby, but there's still the question, what if we don't win? What if we don't get him?'" (A35).

Calvert and her husband began decorating a room for the baby, but stopped because it became too painful when Johnson began threatening to sue for custody. Now Calvert wants to "buy a changing table and finish wallpapering the room with bright Disney characters" (A35). This information makes the Calverts sound like stable, loving parents who have indeed been harmed by the legal battle over the baby created with their genetic material. The most important piece of information provided about Johnson is that she has no genetic link to the child, a fact that the judge will use to deny her any custody rights.

The coverage of the same case presented in the *New York Times* gives greater context to the issues involved. By comparing the Johnson case to another in which a woman past menopause gave birth to a child using a donated egg, reporter Seth Mydans shows us the same contradictory legal situation that feminist commentator Katha Pollitt points out in *The Nation*. Mydans quotes attorney Lori Andrews, author of two books on contract motherhood, "In these two instances we have exactly the same biological situation, yet we *want* different legal results" (emphasis added IV, 6).

Because of the Johnson case, Mydans tells us, the definition of mother has been challenged. He then allows another expert to articulate the problem when he quotes James Nelson of the Hastings Center, a medical ethics research institution. Nelson explains that Judge Parslow's decision, and his comparison of Anna Johnson to a foster parent, "'offers an image of women as interchangeable fetal containers, and [suggests] that when it comes down to it, any womb will do'" (IV, 6).

Mydans warns of the potential for exploitation when he tells the reader that Ramona Ripston, of the American Civil Liberties Union, is concerned about "the possible creation of a breeder class of poor women who 'rent out their wombs' to more affluent women who may seek to avoid a nine-month interruption in their careers" (IV, 6). Mydans allows the administrator of the Center for Surrogate Parenting to rebut this criticism. Polly Craig claims that the "$10,000 fee is too low to serve as the motive for most surrogate mothers," though they may be doing so out of guilt over an abortion (IV, 6). The article closes with Craig claiming that in her program the contract mother bonds with the childless couple rather than the baby. Again we see reference to the characteristic displacement created by these arrangements: the mother-child bond is said to be replaced by the surrogate-sister-in-need bond.

If a contract mother were really seen as simply "a person whose womb was let for rent," then a billboard erected over a Houston freeway in 1993 would not have received the coverage that it did in the *Houston Chronicle*. Advertising herself with the lines "Womb for Rent! Educated, Healthy, Loving Surrogate Mother Available," an anonymous woman declared through an attorney that she wished to finance her Ph.D. by renting out her womb (Warren "Sign" 1A). The incident received front page coverage as a rather humorous affair with a headline that read "Sign gives pregnant pause" (1A). The woman is characterized by her attorney as "'substantial, well-educated, . . . with a nice personality and a stable personality profile—not a nut case in any way, shape or form'" (Broach qtd. in Warren 12A). She describes herself as having a healthy "'environment of the womb'" (qtd. in Lenhart 17A) and both she and her attorney believe that she deserves a special premium in her compensation because of her unique approach (Warren "Sign" 12A).

Several days after the billboard went up, the identity of the woman was discovered, and this discovery put an entirely different twist on the story. In a follow-up article, the reader learns that "[t]he woman who advertised her womb for rent on a roadside billboard has been indicted on federal charges of mail fraud and money laundering and is fighting felony charges of writing hot checks in Louisiana" (Warren and Sablatura 1A). The woman was also arrested in 1983 after allegedly shooting her first husband (16A). (The charges were dropped and she collected $2 million in life insurance (Warren "Womb" 11A).) Her second husband turns out to be Roger Broach, the attorney handling her womb rental campaign (Warren "Surrogate" 1A). The writer reports that the woman lives "from scam to scam," and these scams are usually of a medical nature (Warren and Sablatura 1A). Once these discoveries are made, the woman's alleged criminal past becomes the main focus of the story; the ethical problem raised by her advertisement of a body part for rent is never questioned in any way.

The final treatment of this case shows that while reproductive capacities may be becoming compartmentalized, our expectation that women should be pure, pious, and submissive has not changed. After painting the womb renter as a brazen cheat, who enjoys taking advantage of others, the reporter ends the story with a quote from the attorney who was representing her first husband in divorce proceedings against her. "That's probably one of the last wombs you want to use" (Sloan qtd. in Warren "Womb" 11A). Apparently we do believe that women like Anna Johnson do more than just provide a biological form of foster care. The implication is that the grade or quality of the womb has a direct bearing on the quality of the child produced therein. Will we read news articles in the future reporting that parents are suing their contract mothers because their children turned out to be criminals?

All of the above images of women—as yearning for motherhood, the ultimate expression of domesticity; as pious and pure in their technologically-assisted pregnancies; and as submissive in their willingness to give up their children—are the rough material for the depictions we saw in the other periodicals. The news media provide the same raw characterizations of the fertility specialists as well. *Time* magazine's publisher may have initiated the media representation of "the-gynecologist-as-the-right-hand-of-God" when in 1978 he called Patrick Steptoe the "cloistered doctor" (Meyers 2). In the cover story printed on Louise Joy Brown before she was born, the doctor is described as "a highly respected gynecologist" ("The First" 59), a fine organist, and an "impeccable dresser" who likes cricket (62). A colleague interviewed for the piece says he is "'a man of character and determination'" (62). Similarly, the reader discovers that Steptoe's partner Edwards is father of five daughters, "no less accomplished in his own field, . . . and just as dedicated" (62).

Newsweek's coverage is not much different: "Steptoe, 65, is a flamboyant and somewhat mysterious figure" with "an unquestioned reputation in gynecology" (Gwynne 67). The Browns are thanking God and Steptoe equally for their child, but give credit for her birth to Steptoe: "'The man who deserves all the praise is Mr. Steptoe" says John Brown, who is obviously in awe of the doctor: "'What a man to be able to do such a wonderful thing'" (Brown qtd. in Gwynne 69).

Newsweek also reports favorably on Howard and Georgeanna Jones, of the Norfolk Institute. They are portrayed not only as the preeminent American IVF experts, but also as the caring couple who had already "grandparented" eight children into the world as early as 1982 (Keerdoja 110). The atmosphere at their clinic is comforting, like "'group therapy'" says one patient who describes the Joneses as very "'sensitive to the women's anxiety'" (Fleck qtd. in Keerdoja 110). Howard Jones is always available for consultation and Georgeanna Jones "'holds your hand during most procedures'" (Fleck qtd. in Keerdoja 110). A 1997 article in the *New York Times* with the telling title "The Gods of Fertility" demonstrates two of the country's leading fertility specialists in action. Drs. Mark Sauer and Zev Rosenwaks explain how they decide some of the ethical dilemmas that are inevitable in their field. Sauer is in the process of deciding to do a special in vitro procedure for a man infected with HIV. Based on the assumption that a single sperm taken from the man will not transmit the virus to his wife or child, Sauer says "it's not fair to deny them that opportunity, if we can do it with informed consent" (qtd. in Bruni B1). Rosenwaks explains why he broke his own ruled regarding age limits to do an in vitro procedure for a 45-year-old woman who lost her family in the Holocaust. The woman felt quite strongly about continuing her family line and Dr. Rosenwaks understood this concern "on a deep level" (Bennet qtd. in Bruni B6).

The news magazines do provide some negative images of doctors as well, and these sound remarkably like the nineteenth-century depictions of the medical quack we read about in chapter two.

Newsweek's coverage of the Del Zio case pits the doctors who destroyed the fertilized egg against Shettles, who conducted the experiment. The "experts" claimed that Shettles was not only unqualified, but the "procedures had been so slipshod that, had the fertilized egg been implanted, Mrs. Del Zio would have contracted peritonitis and perhaps died" (Footlick 70). Shettles is characterized as "controversial" and though the reporter explains that Shettles is an acknowledged pioneer in the field, he also informs the reader that the doctor was demoted to the admissions desk (70).

Time editor Philip Elmer-DeWitt explains that there are horror stories about the "poorly trained physician" who schedules fertility treatments and invasive surgery on women without first checking sperm counts ("Making Babies" 63). This is the technological equivalent of prescribing "oil of savin." In the same article, Dr. Richard Marrs, defined as an infertility expert, scoffs at those who do fertility work for selfish reasons: "'They pick up infertility because it's easier than delivering babies at 3 a.m.'" (63).

Elmer-DeWitt profiles one such "quack," Dr. Cecil Jacobson, a fertility expert who was accused of using his own sperm to inseminate patients. This errant doctor is also portrayed as an egotist. He reportedly tells his patients: "'God doesn't give you babies, I do'" ("The Cruelest" 27). Elmer-DeWitt points out that "[t]he disturbing case of Dr. Jacobson underscores a problem that has plagued the booming field of infertility medicine. Doctors can claim to be experts on the basis of scant experience or training. There is no board certification and little regulation" (27). By making a distinction between the "true" expert and the quack, this news coverage succeeds at legitimizing fertility practices, so long as they are performed by a recognized authority. This is precisely the function of the medical case history we saw working to establish basic gynecological practice in the nineteenth century.

If technology can be harmful in the hands of an alleged medical quack and beneficial in the hands of an expert, then the technology itself can be presented as having neutral value. Some of the news coverage aims at this type of presentation, while more recent coverage has developed a more critical focus.

Time's cover story on Louise Joy Brown indicates that while some thought the claim of a test-tube birth was a hoax, others "heralded the coming birth as a miracle of modern medicine" ("The First" 58). The miracle metaphor, combined with the following characterization of the birth as a "scientifically assisted blessed event" (58), reinforces the association of science with God's purposes. Matt Clark, writing for *Newsweek* makes the same linguistic association: "Today they are *blessed* with a broad new array of medical possibilities, . . . " (emphasis added 102). He adds the magical allusion as well when he describes "the magic of microsurgery" (103) and announces that "[i]n vitro fertilization is the most spectacular development of all" (103).

Both *Time* and *Newsweek* include a good share of criticism for IVF-related procedures. *Time*'s line-up includes Dr. John Marshall, head of obstetrics and gynecology at Los Angeles County's Harbor General Hospital who says that "'[t]he potential for misadventure is unlimited,'" (59) and James Watson, Nobel Laureate, who predicts bad scenarios with what is now known as gestational surrogacy (61). *Newsweek* includes comments from Father William Smith who "fear[s] that we may be slipping away from doctoring the patient to doctoring the race" (qtd. in Gwynne 67) and biochemist Dr. Leon Kass: "Perhaps a wise society would say to infertile couples: 'We understand your sorrow, but it might be better not to go ahead and do this'" (qtd. in Gwynne 71). For balance, science writer Isaac Asimov is quoted taking the neutral stance, and claiming that governments and people are responsible for how we use the technology that scientists develop (71).

Even if the experts perceive the technology as neutral, they critique it for its potential role in enabling women to misuse it in immoral—or at least unfeminine ways. A *New York Times* article tells of the birth of four babies within a ten-day period, all created from the genetic material of a Venezuelan couple (Lawson 1:1). In this article medical ethicists express their concerns that women will abuse reproductive services by hiring contract mothers simply to avoid the inconvenience of pregnancy. To counter these concerns, fertility experts say they will not perform the procedure unless it is medically necessary (1:24). This view implies that women place very little value on pregnancy, when the evidence suggests just the opposite. The women who volunteer for these procedures do so to achieve pregnancy first and foremost. They usually resort to contractual arrangements only after they have exhausted all other avenues—including exhausting their own physical pain and endurance thresholds.

Another example of this distrust, not of the technology but of women's motivations for using it, appears in a *Newsweek* article about the Nobel Sperm Bank. In this small profile, the mother of the first baby born from Nobel Prize winning sperm is accused of being a child abuser. She has lost custody of two other children, the writer explains, and she is a convicted felon who was paroled shortly after the sperm bank opened. Apparently, she and her second husband wanted a genius child and plan to begin their daughter's training as early as possible ("The Sperm" 24). In response to the controversy caused by this woman's background, a spokesman for the sperm bank says they will now ask about the criminal records of women who seek sperm (24).

Another interesting feature of the news media's depiction of reproductive technology is that doctors working with genetic materials tend to anthropomorphize and sexualize the gametes and their functions. In a 1991 article Elmer-DeWitt describes GIFT, one of the latest technologies: "[H]e simply loaded the sperm and eggs . . . into a fine pipette and inserted them into the Fallopian tube, where he hoped they would *take care of business by themselves*" (emphasis added 61). The implication is that the egg and sperm simply needed to be properly "introduced." Another specialist explains that nutrients are added to eggs after removal because "'[y]ou don't want the eggs to suspect they are out of the body'" (Brackett qtd in "The First" 66). It's nice to know that some doctors think of eggs as brainy, but of course Elmer-DeWitt characterizes them as sexy as well: "only eggs that emitted the 'come hither' message were successfully fertilized" ("Making Babies" 61). In a 1996 article on some of the latest technologies, Dr. John Buster, director of Baylor's Division of Reproductive Endocrinology and Infertility, discusses the "hormonal conversation" that the uterus and the egg engage in: "'The uterus is smart,' Buster said. 'It will not allow anything less than perfect. It's awesome how this works'" (4E).

The news coverage also includes specific reporting of religious views of reproductive technologies. Lesley Brown's by-now-familiar rationale takes on the linguistic features of prayer when she says "'we just had to pray to God to give our thanks. It seemed right and natural'" ("To Fool" 69). This sentence closely resembles a prayer in the Catholic Church service: "It is right to give him thanks and praise." A Jewish authority who disagrees with the rabbi quoted earlier explains his approval of reproductive technologies: "'When nature does not permit conception, it is desirable to try to outwit nature. The Talmud teaches that God desires man's cooperation'" (Siegel qtd. in "To Fool" 69). The Roman Catholic Church, however, presents a consistent point of view: "'[I]nterference with nature is not acceptable' in any form" ("To Fool" 69).

The *Houston Chronicle* coverage of the 62-year-old Italian woman who gave birth recently also included the Catholic Church's response. In a follow-up to the "Mama mia" story, the author explains that Dr. Antinori's creation of "granny pregnancies [has] unleashed an ethical storm in Roman Catholic Italy, where a lack of legislation has made the country a magnet for post-menopausal women who want to have children" ("Vatican" 16A). The Church's position on the event is that the woman has committed a "morally reprehensible act" (16A).

The status of the products of all of this technology—both the embryo and the child—is the subject of a great deal of discussion and debate in the news media. Because of events like Jerry Hall's cloning of an embryo in 1993, the cloning of Dolly the lamb in 1997, Britain's 1996 embryo destruction, and the birth of the McCaughey septuplets, the news has turned its attention to questions like the following: What is the moral status of pregnancy reduction? "Do embryos, frozen or thawed, have a constitutional right to life? How much manipulation of genetic material will society be willing to permit?" (Elmer-DeWitt "Making Babies" 58). A situation in which a couple with frozen embryos died in an airplane crash provoked the question: "Does an orphaned embryo have a right to a womb?" (Press 54). In anticipation of future cases, Harvard lawyer William Curran speculates that children with deformities caused by reproductive technology will file malpractice suits against their parents (Gwynne 72).

One case that brought the status of the embryo into court, and which provided the impetus for Allegretti's comments in *America*, was argued in Tennessee in 1989. Junior and Mary Sue Davis, sued each other for custody of the seven frozen embryos they had on reserve. She wanted to implant them and he wanted to stop her from having his child. She argued that the embryos were alive and that she should have the right to carry them and he argued that the embryos were property. The judge awarded custody to the woman based on the premise that human life begins at conception and that implantation would serve the "best interest of these children" (May 1A).

By determining that the embryos were children, the judge added another kink to the ongoing debate over abortion. This is the first issue covered in a *Los Angeles Times* article on the case. Kate Michelman, of the National Abortion Rights Action League, is quoted as saying that the judge's decision is "ludicrous" and has "dangerous implications for reproductive freedom in America" (A1, A19). Additional issues addressed in the article include whether the husband would be required to pay child support should his ex-wife succeed in carrying any of the embryos to term, and what would happen to the rest of them should she decide to stop trying. The author also quotes a biomedical ethicist from USC, Alexander M. Capron, who claims that the ruling poses a contradiction. If the embryos are to be treated as human beings, then how do we determine that each receives fair treatment? If one is picked over another for implantation, how is that decision to be made (A19)?

The case was appealed by Junior Davis and the appeals court overturned the lower court's decision ("Divorced" A20). By giving the Davises joint custody, the court made a Solomon-like decision that essentially said to the couple "You created the problem, now you resolve it." Mary Sue Davis tried to donate the embryos to a fertility clinic, but that attempt was also blocked by her ex-husband.

Cryo-preservation techniques have resulted in the storage worldwide of thousands of embryos with uncertain legal status. Britain passed a law in 1991 that embryos could not be stored longer than five years without the consent of the "owners" of the genetic material. The result of this law was that in 1996 some 3300 embryos were destroyed in British fertility clinics. The housecleaning stirred a heated debate over the practice of storing embryos. Several articles appeared on the subject, many of them reporting on religious figures' reactions to the event. A *Houston Chronicle* article quotes the Vatican calling the destruction a "'pre-natal massacre'" and England's Catholic leader, Cardinal Basil Hume, calling it an "appalling dilemma" (Johnson 20A).

An even more provocative practice is the creation of embryos for "adoption." When clinics have leftover genetic material, they mix and match to create "pre-fab" embryos that couples can choose for reduced rates. A *New York Times* article by Gina Kolata describes the practice in detail. Kolata asks: "Is there something chilling about the idea of making embryos on speculation and selecting egg and sperm donors according to their looks, education, and ethnicity?" (A34). The author allows law professor Lori B. Andrews to answer the question for her: "'It does seem like a supermarket approach to embryos'" (A34). The view of a couple who selected some of these embryos is also heard in the article. For the Butlers, the ready-made embryos were a last chance at parenthood. They had already exhausted their money trying to use their own genetic material. "'It's an adoption, but we have control.' Mrs. Butler said. 'We don't have to worry about the birth mother changing her mind. We don't have to worry that she'll take drugs while she's pregnant'" (qtd. in Kolata A34).

In October of 1993, and in February of 1997, two events occurred that crystallized concerns about the status of the embryo created by in vitro technologies. In 1993, a scientist in Washington successfully cloned a human embryo in his laboratory and in 1997 Scottish scientists announced the successful cloning of a lamb from an adult cell. Many of the ethical issues related to in vitro that have remained dormant till now are provoked by the idea of cloning. Because it could be used to reproduce identical copies of a host, cloning threatens our sense of individuality; and certainly the myth of the individual is a unique and important part of American culture.

A *New York Times* article by Gina Kolata reprinted in the *Houston Chronicle* focuses on some of the ethical issues. As soon as the author tells us what happened and where, she explains that the experiment "opens a range of practical and ethical questions" (4A). The example she cites is that while one embryo is allowed to be born, another can be frozen and then used years later to create a younger, identical twin to the first.

The doctor who produced the cloned embryo, Dr. Jerry L. Hall, did so in an attempt to create more embryos for in vitro fertilization. He declined to comment for the article. Instead the reporter quotes the often-interviewed Arthur Caplan who says that cloning is "morally and legally of concern" because it is fairly easy to do (4A).

The *New York Times* reporter just touches the tip of the controversy, and where she leaves off, both *Time* and *Newsweek* take over. In an article titled "Clone Hype," *Newsweek* author Jerry Adler comments on the newsworthiness of cloning by calling a story that puts the words human and clone together "one of the most sought-after coups of 20th century journalism" (60). Adler explains that the *New York Times* article mistakenly implied that human embryos were being routinely cloned in laboratories. This erroneous report created an hysterical reaction involving bioethicists and demonstrators. Adler downplays the experiment performed by Dr. Jerry Hall when he writes: "This [the reaction] was all to the bemusement of Dr. Jerry Hall and his colleagues at George Washington University, who had set out merely to find a more efficient technique for in vitro fertilization, and weren't sure they had achieved even that much" (60).

While it is true that a *New York Times* headline announcing the advent of human cloning would be sure to set off a passionate reaction, Adler's statement depicts the event quite casually. He also interviews Dr. Arthur Caplan, but he selects a quote that implies a very different attitude for Caplan than in the previous article: "I've never seen anything like this gut, visceral fear of cloning,. . . . People are afraid of it because they don't know anything about it" (60). This quote makes it appear as though Caplan approves of the procedure, but if we look closely at his quotes in both articles, it is not apparent how he really feels.

The overall impression created by Adler's article is that Dr. Hall's work is not earth-shattering and that any anti-cloning reaction is extreme. He labels one cloning opponent—Jeremy Rifkin—a "biotech gadfly," and explains that Hall's work was done for the best of reasons: to "improve the chances of success with in-vitro fertilization . . . " (61). This statement indicates acceptance of the technology in general, and of the goal of having several identical embryos to implant. Adler does acknowledge that some frightening scenarios are plausible—such as using a clone for organ donation, or selling the cloned embryos of sports figures—but finally he says that we should get on with the business of designing some regulations so that "scientists [can] get on with work that may save some lives or bring wanted life into the world" (62).

Time magazine's coverage of this event demonstrates a more critical attitude. Philip Elmer-DeWitt gives a full view of the problems cloning could create. He reports on several potential abuses suggested by the much-interviewed Arthur Caplan: catalogues of cloned children, couples setting clones aside in case a child dies; women giving birth to their own twins, and finally, clones used for organ donation.

Elmer-DeWitt does not stop with the ethical dilemmas suggested by cloning, however, he also acknowledges that in vitro fertilization has already created dilemmas of its own. He quotes IVF experts who are angry about Hall's experiment because it placed IVF in the public eye. Hall has opened the proverbial "can of worms," forcing the public to pay attention to reproductive technology and the questions it poses (70). Some of these current questions include the status of the some 10,000 embryos that are currently in frozen storage in the United States

(69). Clones or not, these embryos can be sold, thawed out, lost in implantation, argued over in custody suits, and used for genetic material. Children are already being conceived to serve as bone marrow donors for older siblings (Dowling 80).

Elmer-DeWitt also refers to Jeremy Rifkin, but instead of calling him a gadfly he gives him a title, "founder of the Foundation on Economic Trends, a biotechnology-watchdog group in Washington" (69). Using his title gives Rifkin more credibility and calling him a watchdog makes him much more palatable than a gadfly. Rifkin is concerned about government abuse of cloning, similar to that of the government in the novel *Brave New World*, but Elmer-DeWitt downplays potential government abuse and instead quotes George Annas, a Boston University medical ethicist: "'But we're in America, where we have the private market. We don't need government to make the nightmare scenario come true'" (69). The inclusion of this comment indicates that Elmer-DeWitt takes the possible repercussions of cloning more seriously than his *Newsweek* counterparts. On the issue of regulation, he says that establishing a national bioethical policy board "had better be done quickly" (69-70) because Hall claims his cloning technique could be functional within a couple of years. Elmer-DeWitt ends by saying of technology that "[t]he time to discuss whether it is right or wrong is before it has been put to use, not after" (70).

These predictions about cloning and the calls for ethical debate were prophetic given the rate at which cloning techniques have been developed and improved. Four short years later we meet Dolly the lamb, and a barrage of media coverage arguing both for and against a practice that promises to become science fact rather than fiction in the immediate future. *Newsweek*'s extensive coverage of this event labels human cloning the "forbidden fruit of biotechnology" (Begley 54). The author's attitude towards the scientists involved and her characterization of their intentions reflects an increasing distrust of our scientific leaders. Begley writes that scientists' surprise over Dolly's creation was "somewhat hollow" after the cloning attempt by Hall in 1993. Her sarcastic portrayal of the Roslin biotechnologists responsible for Dolly reveals the fear that a procedure such as cloning inspires: "The Roslin scientists had no sooner trotted out Dolly than they assured everyone who asked that no one would ever, *ever*, apply the technology that made Dolly to humans. Pressed to answer whether human cloning was next, scientists prattled on about how immoral, illegal, and pointless such a step would be" (56).

Time magazine's coverage of the cloning includes a wryly humorous discussion by Jeffrey Kluger that profiles several potential cloning clinic customers. They include the grieving parents of a child with leukemia who want a clone for a bone marrow transplant, the wealthy industrialist who wants an heir to the family business, and the terminally ill physics laureate who can't bear the idea of leaving the world without his brilliance. The despot is mentioned as well, thinking of cloning as a way to ensure his power over his little country. After painting these uncomfortable scenarios, Kluger allows several bioethicists to speak. Most oppose the idea of cloning humans, but they also do not see how the science involved can be stopped. Art Caplan's prediction that a cloned infant will be born in the next seven years appears at the end of the piece, along with Kluger's recommendation that "science had better get its ethical house in order quickly" (72).

Nearly a year after the Scottish breakthrough, The *New York Times*' Gina Kolata reports that the possibility of human cloning has already become somewhat accepted by fertility clinics. The Federal Government, which does not support human cloning research, is funding cloning research in monkeys. Law professor Lori Andrews is quoted describing the stages the public goes through when advances are made in reproductive techniques: "from 'horrified negation' to 'negation without horror' to 'slow and gradual curiosity, study, evaluation, and finally a very slow but steady acceptance'" (A24). According to Andrews, the slow but steady acceptance stage has already been reached on the subject of human cloning. The final word on the subject is from a fertility expert who is already experimenting with nuclear transfer: "'The fact is that, in America, cloning may be bad but telling people how they should reproduce is worse'" (Willadsen qtd. in Kolata A24).

This same ethical dilemma was also played out over another 1997 news event: the birth of septuplets in Iowa. On November 19, Bobby and Kenny McCaughey became the parents of the world's first surviving septuplets and they also sparked a national debate over the safety of fertility drugs, the ethics of fertility practices such as pregnancy reduction (killing several fetuses in a multiple pregnancy so that the others have a better chance of survival), and the wisdom of choosing to maintain a multiple pregnancy despite the great odds against the babies' survival and health. The headlines were often humorous and catchy: "It's a boy, girl, boy, girl, boy, girl, oh boy!" (Pressley A1), "In Iowa, the Birth of a Nation" ("In Iowa" 66), "The Magnificent Seven" (McCormick and Kantrowitz 58), and "It's a Miracle" (Lemonick 34). The discussion, however, was frequently quite critical, ranging from questions about whether the fertility specialist who treated Bobby McCaughey warned her about the potential for a multiple pregnancy to complaints that the state of Iowa was showering gifts on the family while ignoring the fate of the many homeless children in the state. In the midst of the coverage about the generosity of various corporations that offered donations, someone asked why an African-American Washington D.C. couple who had given birth to sextuplets had been ignored. Corporate America scrambled to make up for the "oversight" and those babies too are assured a comfortable future.

The news media coverage of reproductive technology is important because it provides its reader with a first glance at these practices. When a reporter uses language like "scientifically assisted blessed event" and calls in vitro births miracles, he or she introduces the miracle metaphor into the cultural text. The metaphor can then be appropriated by other periodical media. The analysis of the women's magazine coverage of reproductive technology shows how such practices can be portrayed through the framework provided by this type of metaphor. When a reporter interviews and quotes experts who denounce IVF-related practices, he or she also introduces the critical view into the cultural text. The newspaper critique motivates the more penetrating debate over reproductive technology found most often in the commentary journal.

NOTES

1. I recognize that locating gynecology at the breakfast table may also call up images of the pre-Roe v. Wade gynecological kitchen table.

CHAPTER SIX

Gynecology in Dystopia

"Literature is news that stays." (Ezra Pound)[1]

If the newspaper is the first draft of history, then the novel represents history in one of its most revised drafts. Because of the genre in which he or she works, the novelist is able to refine a representation of reality in a text that can both delight and instruct at the same time. With complete control over the "facts" of the case, the novelist can manipulate events and characters to convey social messages and create emotional reactions. The reader expects the novelist to create a consistent and predictable world within the boundaries set by the novel, recognizing that while the novelistic world is fictitious it is drawn from the "real" one. The novelist working with the gynecological case history can combine the same elements of fantasy and commentary we saw pulled together in the news media, but this combination is a homogenous one, used to present a consistent point of view.

In *Abortion, Choice, and Contemporary Fiction*, Judith Wilt begins her discussion of the novelistic treatment of abortion with case histories: "[f]or lives, actual experiences, are surely the basis of art; and the fact is that the reality and multiplicity of experience are always in danger of being overwhelmed by, hyperordered by art" (xii). The three novelists for this coda to the discussion of the periodical media have been chosen precisely because their art has not overwhelmed the reality and multiplicity of experience. Novelists Aldous Huxley, Margaret Atwood, and Sarah Bird use their fictitious gynecological case histories to reintroduce some of the problems that have been left out of previous accounts. Because *Brave New World*, *The Handmaid's Tale*, and *The Mommy Club* hold our cultural attitudes and their resulting scientific technologies up to scrutiny, their fictions are in a sense more realistic than those supposedly "real life" accounts we encounter in the news media and their fictional fantasies are very different from the ones crafted for the women's magazines.

Writing about horror and fantasy, Rosemary Jackson explains that literary fantasy exposes that which has been repressed to the unconscious:

> Un-doing those unifying structures and significations upon which social order depends, fantasy functions to subvert and undermine cultural stability. It proposes what Cixous calls 'a subtle invitation to transgression' by exposing the relative and arbitrary nature of those 'responses' [which men make] to death: ideological institutions, religion, politics.' (69-70)

The (bordering on) fantastic worlds created by Huxley and Atwood and the distinctly real world created by Bird expose the ideologies that make both scientific reproduction and the exploitation of women in the service of this technology possible. The rigidly stratified society that has been genetically engineered in Huxley's *Brave New World* parodies the socio-economic boundaries that already structure our culture, and the "two-legged womb" (146) status of Offred and her peers in *The Handmaid's Tale* illuminates the attitude toward women that underlies the popularity of the surrogacy industry. The stifling control that Hillary Goettler tries to exercise over Trudy, her contract mother, in *The Mommy Club* is an example of the business-like attitude that existing surrogacy arrangements attempt to apply to the complex emotional and physical phenomenon of conception and birth. These authors have created societies that come, not from the range of the remotely possible, but from the range of the probable, based on social structures and attitudes that are already in play.

In a discussion of modern satirists, Stephen Jay Greenblatt explains that Huxley's novel reflects his concern about the social conditions of the 1920s:

> *Brave New World*, like Orwell's *1984*, is primarily concerned not with what will happen in the future but what is happening to mankind now. A futuristic detail like the hatching of babies from bottles, for example, is less an interesting scientific speculation than an ironic

> comment on the dissociation of sexuality and childbirth and on the ultimate artificiality of the inhabitants of our brave new world. (96)

The last sentence of this quote from Greenblatt's 1965 essay is somewhat ironic. The technologies of in vitro fertilization and contractual motherhood had not yet been realized, and the factory production of children did seem only a futuristic detail. Today, barely 30 years later, these technologies are real. By the turn of the century, if the artificial womb has been perfected, Huxley's "Central London Hatchery and Conditioning Centre" could cease to be a thing of fiction. But Greenblatt is absolutely correct in pointing out that Huxley is commenting on the dissociation of sexuality and childbirth and the artificiality which were characteristic of the 1920s and 30s. These characteristics made the medical technology not only possible, but acceptable.

In *The Handmaid's Tale*, Atwood expresses her concern that the present will shape the future in ways we have not examined. "By envisioning an appalling future already implicit in the contemporary world, Atwood condemns just those present propensities that make a Gilead possible . . . " (Davidson 113). All of the elements of Gilead exist today, and Atwood is commenting on the attitudes and belief systems that allow women to be exploited as walking wombs or as Offred describes herself, as "national resource[s]" (85). These are the attitudes that make the practice of contract motherhood acceptable, even attractive for some.

By drawing on recent surrogacy situations, Sarah Bird creates a couple in *The Mommy Club* that is representative of the stereotypical consumer of the surrogacy industry. Trudy, the contract mother, has been drafted into service as an incubator by a pair of wealthy, attractive "yuppies" who have decided that it is time to reproduce. Hillary Goettler, the wife, illustrates all the elite behaviors worried over by commentators who believe that women will misuse surrogacy arrangements. She is visibly relieved to find out that she is infertile because just the thought of what pregnancy would do to her body makes her cringe. Victor Goettler is along for the ride, though he finds the human part of the equation distinctly uncomfortable. Trudy characterizes his reaction to her pregnancy: "He treats me as if I might be carrying a thermonuclear device instead of his child" (67). Together, the Goettlers try to control every moment of Trudy's pregnancy. They move her into their house and monitor every morsel she puts in her mouth:

> "Just think," Hillary slides my napkin out and pulls it across my lap. "The baby is going to get *double* nutritional benefits from this meal." . . . "Well, dig in." Hillary stands behind me and waits. I fiddle with my fork and take deep breaths through my mouth so that none of the liver smell will reach my stomach. (Bird's emphasis 18)

By painting a much less than flattering picture of the Goettlers, Bird presents strong criticism of the attitudes held by many of the couples who pursue surrogacy. Trudy is also everything a contract mother should not be and is therefore extremely susceptible to exploitation. She is too old, flighty, emotionally unbalanced, and acting as a surrogate for all the wrong reasons, but she is also convenient for Hillary and Victor, who have a strong (and ultimately unfounded) faith in their ability to control the situation.

In previous chapters we have seen how language can be pressed into the service of science and technology. In this chapter, we will see the authors depict worlds in which this function of language is carried out, and at the same time called into question. The purpose of these novels is to subvert that relationship with language, using the language of the novel to pierce through the ideological norms we have come to accept. In his introduction to the 1946 edition of *Brave New World*, Aldous Huxley writes:

> The greatest triumphs of propaganda have been accomplished, not by doing something, but by refraining from doing. Great is truth, but still greater, from a practical point of view, is silence about truth. By simply not mentioning certain subjects, by lowering what Mr. Churchill calls an "iron curtain" between the masses and such facts or arguments as the local political bosses regard as undesirable, totalitarian propagandists have influenced opinion much more effectively than they could have done by the most eloquent denunciations, the most compelling of logical rebuttals. (xii)

When Huxley's character Helmholtz Watson, whose job it is to write the inane jingles that make up the cultural wisdom of his world, begins to break free from his programming, he says he wants to write words that do more than just sound good. He wants to create "[w]ords [that] can be like X-rays, if you use them properly—they'll go through anything. You read and you're pierced" (47). Helmholtz' problem is that he must write about nothing and he can't use his X-ray words on nothing. When he does experiment by writing a poem about loneliness, he is immediately reported by his students; the poem is one of the reasons for his subsequent exile. In this brave new world, creative vision is not tolerated because it challenges the stability of the culture. In this world, language is a tool of repression rather than expression.

Huxley understands the great power that words wield. In *Brave New World*, words are used to engineer programmed responses to feelings. The members of this society are first genetically engineered and then "hypnopædically" programmed in their sleep with "moral" beliefs intended to help them to achieve stability and happiness. "A gramme is always better than a damn" is Lenina's hypnopædically induced response to Bernard's bad mood (60). She is referring to a gramme of soma, the wonder drug that immediately obliterates any strongly felt emotion. Helmholtz serves as a representative of Huxley in the novel, embodying the choice he must make as an author. He can either parrot the conventional wisdom of his society and remain safely within bounds, or he can look beneath the surface, and by exposing the problems he sees put himself at risk for exile.

Margaret Atwood shares in this role of social examiner. In an interview, she explains "the writer may unconsciously reflect the society, he may consciously examine it and project ways of changing it; and the connection between the writer and society will increase in intensity as the society . . . becomes the 'subject' of the writer" (Atwood qtd. in Rigney 121).

In *The Handmaid's Tale*, the refusal to examine and confront reality has resulted in the country of Gilead. Offred, who represents the twenty-first-century version of "true womanhood" reminisces about her mother, an active protester in her time. To the young Offred, her mother's protests were something to be slightly embarrassed about; they were unnecessary, outdated:

> You young people don't appreciate things, she'd say. You don't know what we had to go through, just to get to where you are. . . . Don't you know how many woman's lives, how many women's *bodies*, the tanks had to roll over just to get that far? (156)

Offred's response to her mother's complaint is to say "[n]ow, Mother, . . . Let's not get into an argument about nothing" (156). When Offred finds herself stripped of economic power after the government is overthrown, she still refuses to take part in the rather weak protests that take place at first. She has her husband and daughter to think of. Instead she retreats to her domestic sphere; she bakes more. The result of this inaction is that the tanks are now rolling over her body and her daughter's. Not only is she conscripted into service as a handmaid (as the pious and pure container for the Commander's seed), but a social structure has been created in which her daughter will be trained to value herself solely by her ability to reproduce: "To 'pay attention', [sic] to look beneath surfaces, to touch and to tell are also imperatives for Offred of *The Handmaid's Tale*. Not paying attention, in fact, is the great fault of Offred's entire society, and the price exacted is the loss of freedom" (Rigney 113).

Language is a weapon of power in Gilead. It is both used and withheld to repress the women of the society. The ritualistic greetings used by the handmaids control how they relate to each other and reinforce their narrowly defined identities as two-legged wombs. "'Blessed be the fruit,' she says to me, the accepted greeting among us./ 'May the Lord open,' I answer, the accepted response" (25). The names bestowed upon them rob them of their former identities and create new ones based solely on their function as submissive and domestic reproductive chattel: Offred, Ofwarren, Ofglen:

> My name isn't Offred, I have another name, which nobody uses now because it's forbidden. I tell myself it doesn't matter, your name is like your telephone number, useful only to others; but what I tell myself is wrong, it does matter. I keep the knowledge of this name like something hidden, some treasure I'll come back to dig up, one day. (108)

For all women in this society, reading and writing have been completely prohibited. The marketing is carried out with small pictographic cards. Offred finds a cushion in her room, the word "Faith" embroidered in faded thread, and she wonders who has overlooked it. In the bottom of her clothes cupboard she finds the Latin phrase "Nolite te bastardes carborundorum;" she imagines her predecessor in the room scratching the phrase into the wood and it becomes a secret slogan left just for her. Offred does not know what it means until later, but she does not need to have meaning ascribed to the individual words for it to have a greater meaning. She has been part of an illicit communication. It means hope. "I pray silently: *Nolite te bastardes carborundorum.* I don't know what it means, but it sounds right, and it will have to do, because I don't know what else I can say to God" (117). Later, she asks the Commander for a translation and realizes that he has probably taught it to the former handmaid. The phrase is a man's phrase, an invented Latin expression that school boys wrote in their books. "Don't let the bastards grind you down" translates the Commander (242). It's a joke he tells her, a joke for schoolboys. It is a cruel joke for the former handmaid whose life has been so conscripted by the patriarchy that her one impotent act of defiance can only be done in the language of her oppressor. She later hangs herself from the chandelier.

The Commander has the power to give language to Offred as a part of a bargain, a bribe for her silence about their illegal meetings in his study. He plays Scrabble with her; he offers her *Vogue* and *Mademoiselle*, even an old *Ms* magazine! She reads them voraciously, these texts she once derided as unworthy of reading. The irony of his offering of these publications can only be fully appreciated after examining the way in which they portray contract motherhood.

Offred herself is a composition, a constructed self. From her new name to her every action, she moves through this new world hiding her former identity. "I wait. I compose myself. My self is a thing I must now compose, as one composes a speech. What I must present is a made thing, not something born" (86). This act of self-composure is itself an act of writing and an act of detachment. To protect what she has left of herself, Offred creates an outer self that can exist as a handmaid and maintains an inner self waiting for the opportunity to gain its freedom.

Offred's true self is preserved in the telling of her story; it is a taped account, but she succeeds in the act of composing. Even this act of defiance is subverted by the "scholarly" discussion that forms the "Historical Notes" section of the novel. This section, which is appended to the tale, is the transcript of the "Twelfth Symposium on Gileadean Studies," held in the year 2195 (379). Gileadean scholars have gathered together for sessions on interpreting the tale and discovering its significance to the Gileadean period, in between attending the nature walk and the "Outdoor Period-Costume Sing-Song" (379). The speaker at this session, Professor Pieixoto, explains how the tapes have been discovered, catalogued and named. The academics have given Offred's story the title, "The Handmaid's Tale," in deference to Geoffrey Chaucer. Pieixoto explains to his audience: "[A]ll puns were intentional, particularly that having to do with the archaic vulgar signification of the word *tail*, that being, to some extent, the bone, as it were, of contention, in that phase of Gileadean society of which our saga treats. (*Laughter, applause*)" (381). Offred has once more been reduced to a "walking womb" in this section that is Atwood's warning to us all about how we choose to make meaning of our history.

In *The Mommy Club* another form of symbolic expression plays a role similar to that of language. Trudy's art is the non-verbal equivalent of the language that is alternately offered to and withheld from Offred. From her gestational chamber at the Goettlers' house, Trudy explains what her art means to her. "I have always had my projects. . . . I've always relied on my art to keep the sand running through the hourglass. That's what I miss the most about living here at the Goettlers, my projects" (10). Her art is her anchor, giving her substance and self-definition. Removing her from her studio is one way in which the Goettlers can appropriate and redefine her for their use, just as denying Offred literacy renders her impotent and redefines her as a stand-in for male potency.

Trudy's works of art are visual puns, her way of making a rather hilarious and biting commentary on the world, and of staying connected—to the world and to herself. When Hillary goes to Trudy's studio to inspect it as a potential incubation site for her child, the projects are everywhere. "Missile toads" are Christmas ornaments: toads dressed in elf outfits sitting on the backs of Minutemen missiles decorated with holly (58). Hillary's response to them is "Ee-yeah. Sounds like fun" (58). Trudy dreams of having Hillary arrange an exhibit for her, while Hillary pokes at the small baby Jesus in a manger scene, who, with ants glued to his back has become the "Anty Christ" (62). Hillary's response to the art is a polite brush-off; her decision about the apartment is that Trudy should move in with her immediately and leave her projects and any identity outside of incubator behind.

Both *Brave New World* and *The Mommy Club*'s use of scientific language to explain reproductive acts imply a critical commentary of the technologies that are at their centers. Huxley's "brave new world" is completely dependent upon the applied sciences of biology, psychology, and sociology. His 1932 vision of reproductive technology comes remarkably close to reality. Human beings are created factory-style; from conception to "decanting" (birth) they are socially, intellectually and emotionally engineered. His depiction of baby "bottling" is colored by the same satiric brush as the rest of the novel; the Director of Hatcheries' scientific explanation of the production of humans shows the danger of valorizing the scientific. He describes Bokanovsky's Process: "'One egg, one embryo, one adult—normality. But a bokanovskified egg will bud, will proliferate, will divide. From eight to ninety-six buds, and every bud will grow into a perfectly formed embryo, and every embryo into a full-sized adult. Making ninety-six human beings grow where only one grew before. Progress'" (3).

The hatchery is science taken to an extreme, every human characteristic is carefully regulated. It is the commentator's nightmare. Mother and Father have become obscene words. Women who have functioning ovaries (most are freemartins), can have "the operation [that is] undergone for the good of Society" (2). The ovary is then kept alive and functioning. Mr. Foster, a bright young Alpha who works in the Fertilizing room brags that the Centre's record for a single ovary is "sixteen thousand and twelve," (5) but he plans to beat the Mombasa record of seventeen thousand:

> "Still," he added, with a laugh (but the light of combat was in his eyes and the lift of his chin was challenging), "still, we mean to beat them if we can. I'm working on a wonderful Delta-Minus ovary at this moment. Only just eighteen months old. Over twelve thousand seven hundred children already, either decanted or in embryo. And still going strong. We'll beat them yet." (5)

This belief in science as progress is what allows the culture to value quantity over quality, and to find in Henry Ford, the inventor of the modern assembly line, a god.

Huxley was extremely concerned with the potential evil that science could do. When Bernard and Lenina visit the savage reservation, they find John Savage, the "natural" son of a Beta minus female named Linda who became accidentally pregnant and was left behind some twenty years before their visit. John and his mother accompany them back to London and it doesn't take long for John to get into trouble. After causing a riot by throwing out the soma intended for a group of Bokanovsky twins, one hundred and sixty-two Deltas, John is brought to Mustapha Mond, the area Controller. In their ensuing conversation, the Controller makes a distinction between pure and applied science. "Every discovery in pure science is potentially subversive; even science must sometimes be treated as the enemy. Yes, even science" (153). He explains that he was once a physicist and, caught doing "a bit of real science" (153), he had to make a choice between being exiled to an island or giving up his science and becoming a Controller. But it is applied science that worries Huxley; in his introduction he warns that the world will lapse into totalitarianism "unless we choose to decentralize and to use applied science, not as the end to which human beings are to be made the means, but as a means to producing a race of free individuals, . . ." (xiv). Jenni Calder explains Huxley's fear of science in more depth:

> For Huxley was profoundly worried about the morality of science, about the fact that knowledge could mean power for evil as well as power for good, that science could destroy as well as discover, and about the fact that the more a small body of highly trained men found out about the way human beings function, the more easily could human beings be controlled. Perhaps his greatest fear was that dangers could occur inadvertently, from the best intentions. (12)

So Huxley worries about how scientific discoveries are applied. These applications must be examined for their moral nature. This is the same warning being sent by many of the commentators discussed in chapter four. It is one we would do well to heed today, as our applications of reproductive technology come dangerously close to Huxley's "brave new world."

The hypnopædic socialization made possible by the application of psychology gives the *Brave New World*'s inhabitants phrases such as the following two exchanged by Bernard and Lenina at the savage reservation: "'But cleanliness is next to fordliness,' she insisted./ 'Yes, and civilization is sterilization,' Bernard went on, concluding on a tone of irony the second hypnopædic lesson in elementary hygiene" (73). "Civilization is sterilization" is certainly an ironic comment. Huxley's fictional society has been sterilized of everything that is essential to humanity: art, passion, pure scientific inquiry. As Greenblatt puts it "[m]an, in using his reason to create the ultimate life of pleasure, has ceased to be man" (97). Is this the logical outcome of trying to manipulate our genetics?

The *Mommy Club*'s depiction of science is no less amusing or sarcastic. Hillary is chosen as the main representative of the reproductive science of our culture, and she is a good choice as she embodies the new lay expert—the woman who, by virtue of her repeated visits to the fertility specialist, has become an authority on conception. The doctors play minor roles: "Tiny, framed portraits of all the tiny babies the doctor had *coaxed* into the world hung in neat rows" (emphasis added 79). The doctors are caricatures: "'Good Old Tee-Time Teeter,' the third nurse says. . . . 'Did I tell you about his latest? Induced after three hours at five centimeters so he could make an eight o'clock tee time. Overdid the pitocin. Uterus set up like concrete and he ended up having to do a section.'" (280)

Hillary, however, is the real thing. She asks Trudy to keep a temperature chart so they can predict her ovulation, but soon starts keeping her own, more detailed one. After one failed attempt at insemination in the doctor's office, (Victor balked at the test tube) Hillary decides they can do it at home. "I went home with Hillary that evening and my body became her own personal laboratory" (84). She first tries pouring Victor's sperm into a cervical cap for Trudy to insert: "'Cervical cap,' she explained. 'I got it as a fallback position. I can see now that the do-it-yourself approach is going to work a lot better for us.' She carefully poured the semen from the party favor cup into the cap. 'Why do we need a middleman? The statistics are just as good without them'"(85). When Trudy proves too clumsy with the cervical cap, they resort to a turkey baster; Hillary is both informed and resourceful.

After a month of trying the baster method, Hillary gets impatient; she wants to do more tests. Trudy describes the humorous scene that follows:

> For most of the month of November daily body temperature readings were enough, then Hillary wanted more. She wanted mucus tests. On the day before Thanksgiving she brought a Bunsen burner, some slides, and counterslips into work. Then, dressed in a Norma Kamali

> cowl-necked black mini accessorized by amber dowry beads from Ghana, she set up shop. (91)

Hillary wants to do more than experiment with Trudy's body; she wants to own the experience. She wants Trudy to have the pain and problems of her pregnancy for her, but she wants the rest for herself. When Hillary discovers that Trudy is thirty-eight and not the twenty-eight she thought her to be, she insists on an amniocentesis. This is just the type of control that Mary Beth Whitehead objected to from the Sterns and which the feminist commentators warn about. Trudy has an ultrasound, and during the procedure Hillary is so intent on seeing "her" baby that Trudy is no longer there in the room. "It startles me when Hillary crowds in to get closer to the screen. She stretches forward even farther and bumps the doctor's hand" (134). In the middle of the procedure, Trudy refuses to have the amnio; she gets up and leaves the doctor's office. Hillary is furious: "'She refuses to have the test. We thought we were getting a twenty-eight-maybe twenty-nine-year-old mother. Trudy's almost thirty-nine and she won't even test for the greatest age-related risk.'"/ Hillary thinks that I am a devious, selfish shit and it suddenly makes not the tiniest bit of difference to me" (137). Hillary can't force Trudy to have the test so she settles into an uncomfortable acceptance of the situation. Later, she reveals the other reason she wanted the test: "For the past month Hillary has been obsessed with decorating the room she is turning into a nursery. . . . She just can't decide on a "motif" and makes occasional references to how much easier the whole process would be if they knew the sex. If I'd had amniocentesis" (177). Science at the service of yuppydom.

The Handmaid's Tale represents a society that has rejected much of its former scientific abilities in favor of a more biblical simplicity. In vitro fertilization and artificial insemination have been ruled out, as well as amniocentesis and chemical assistance at birth:

> What will Ofwarren give birth to? A baby, as we all hope? Or something else, an Unbaby, with a pinhead or a snout like a dog's, or two bodies, or a hole in its heart or no arms, or webbed hands and feet? There's no telling. They could tell once, with machines, but that is now outlawed. What would be the point of knowing anyway? You can't have them taken out; whatever it is it must be carried to term. (143)

This is a society that could use the machines of science to predict the deformities caused by the nuclear accidents that have occurred. Perhaps this world's rejection is partially due to the contribution science has made to the hopeless situation.

The description of Offred's doctor appointment indicates that the science that is still allowed is the depersonalized, object-producing science of today. "At neck level there's another sheet, suspended from the ceiling. It intersects me so that the doctor will never see my face. He deals with a torso only" (78). The doctor is a parody of today's helpful Wizard whose mission is to "help" infertile women to usher new life into the world. Offred has been well-indoctrinated in the virtue of purity. She is shocked when the doctor breaks the rules by lifting the sheet and offering to help her become pregnant. He utters a word that is now outlawed—sterile. "There is no such thing as a sterile man anymore, not officially. There are only women who are fruitful and women who are barren, that's the law" (79). Even in his proposal to her, the doctor continues to see her as an object, a torso to use for his pleasure. Later, when her Commander's wife suggests getting outside "help" to conceive, Offred will pick Nick, the chauffeur, over the cold, objective, yet lascivious doctor.

Brave New World does not have any birth scenes because there are no mothers; we are not even treated to a "decanting." Linda is the only mother in the novel. Her life and death are a good indication of what Huxley believed would happen to a culture that separated reproduction from sexuality. Ashamed of her motherhood, she is forced to remain on the reservation: "'Turned into a savage,' she shouted. 'Having young ones like an animal. . . If it hadn't been for you, I might have gone to the Inspector, I might have got away. But not with a baby. That would have been too shameful'" (85). She becomes an alcoholic to numb the pain, and when she returns to London a social outcast, she becomes a somaholic. "[N]obody had the smallest desire to see Linda. To say one was a mother—that was past a joke; it was an obscenity" (102-103). She goes on a permanent soma holiday and in a very short time the drug kills her.

Lenina, on the other hand, is an example of what happens to a woman when her childbearing function is removed. She is a permanent child in a society where everyone owns everyone and all are sexually available to each other. Though she has fallen in love with John, she is not emotionally equipped to deal with her feelings. She frets and sighs and finally, after taking some soma, gets up her nerve to go tell him how she feels. To her surprise he is also in love with her, but his definition of love is too different from hers. He rejects the purely sexual, wanting something deeper; he wants to do something to prove his worth to her. The only reaction she knows how to have is sexual. She pulls her clothes off and comes towards him, offering herself. John's reaction is to retreat, quoting Shakespeare. "'The strongest oaths are straw to the fire i' the blood. Be more abstemious, or else. . . '" (131). But the full measure of Linda's emotional depth is represented by the only poetry she knows: "'Hug me till you drug me, . . . '" (131). The love scene she has been anticipating disintegrates into a confrontation, with the Savage resorting to violence to spurn her advances.

The other two novels have birth scenes, and in both, the baby is taken from its mother. In both, the child has been created for someone else and the birth mother's role is down-played and devalued. In *The Handmaid's Tale*, Ofwarren's labor is the beginning of a birth celebration, attended by all of the handmaids and wives in the district. Warren's wife mimics the birth; the other wives assist her just as the handmaids assist Ofwarren. "A small thin woman, she lies on the floor, in a white cotton nightgown, her graying hair spreading like mildew over the rug; they massage her tiny belly, just as if she's really about to give birth herself" (150).

When Ofwarren is ready to "deliver" the child, the wife takes her position on the Birthing Stool. Its double seating arrangement allows the wife to frame the handmaid's body and appropriate her labor; just as she attends the monthly "rape" ceremony as the symbolic wife. Once the baby is born, it is the Commander's wife who is tucked into the bed, with the baby in her arms. "The Commander's wife looks down at the baby as if it's a bouquet of flowers: something she's won, a tribute" (163). In a final act of possession, the Commander's wife names the baby.

A month or two later, Offred sees Ofwarren at a "Salvaging," the brutal ceremony in which the handmaids are allowed to commit a cathartic murder. She observes that Ofwarren is no longer with the wife of Warren and that she has been re-posted. It is too soon for Ofwarren to have been moved and Offred speculates that something has gone wrong with her breast milk. "That would be the only reason they'd move her, unless there's been a fight over the baby; which happens more than you'd think. Once she had it, she may have resisted giving it up. I can see that" (278). Apparently the handmaids are not always perfectly submissive about giving their children away. This comment also acknowledges the grief that the handmaids experience when their babies are taken from them. But Offred's grief over losing her own daughter, which permeates her story, is the best indicator of the emotional cost the handmaid is forced to pay:

> I would come up through a roaring and confusion, like surf boiling. I can remember feeling quite calm. I can remember screaming, it felt like screaming though it may have been only a whisper, *Where is she? What have you done with her?*
>
> They showed me a picture of her, standing outside on a lawn, her face a closed oval. Her light hair was pulled back tight behind her head. Holding her hand was a woman I didn't know. She was only as tall as the woman's elbow.
>
> You've killed her, I said. (51-52)

Offred's daughter has been re-possessed and her body has been "commandeered" by a society whose system is set up to separate the functions of childbirth and mothering, except for the very poor—the "Econowives." "These women are not divided into functions. They have to do everything; if they can" (32).

In *The Mommy Club*, Trudy's pregnancy is also something to be re-possessed. She and Hillary attend childbirth classes together. Hillary mimics her symptoms. Their instructor explains that the skin stretching over her stomach makes Trudy itch and Hillary scratches her own stomach. Then Hillary asks about headaches and insomnia. "Rachel looks at me sympathetically, as if Hillary were asking all these questions on my behalf" (220). This appropriation of her pregnancy irritates Trudy. "I am pregnant. Not Hillary. Me. I am the one having a baby. Not Hillary. Me" (222). But it is Hillary, not Trudy whose symptoms are acknowledged and who is soothed and held by her husband. This lack of human warmth when she needs it the most is what sends Trudy to look for her ex-lover Sinclair.

When her daughter is born, Trudy recognizes that the baby has her dreamer's soul and that the Goettlers are not fit parents for her. "I know this child and I know what she needs. . . . I see that Hillary and Victor will not know how to protect her dreamer's soul any more than Randi and Gordon did mine" (362). Instead Trudy gives her baby to her old teacher, Sister Theonella, who runs an illegal adoption agency, because she does not believe that she is capable of raising her herself—a belief that Hillary has been cultivating for the nine months of her pregnancy. She feels the loss immediately: "I can't believe how my arms could ache from holding something so light. . . . I start to scream, to stop her, but still my throat doesn't work. I listen to the snuffling, mewling baby sounds recede down the hall, then the ping of the elevator, then the doors shutting and my baby is gone forever" (366-367).

Better than any of the "real life" case histories, these stories show the reader the true repercussions of such arrangements. When the Goettlers arrive at the hospital and demand to know where their baby is, they assume from Trudy's pained expression that something is wrong with the baby. It hasn't occurred to them that she would be distressed at having to give up her daughter. Hillary assumes the baby has Down's syndrome, and her reaction confirms Trudy's decision not to allow her to mother the child. "'I told you we shouldn't go ahead without the amnio. I told you the risks'. . . . Worse than death is imperfection" (369). Still, Victor tries weakly to keep their end of the agreement. Trudy's response is similar to the responses contract mothers like Mary Beth Whitehead-Gould have had to their real life situations. "'Yes, but the person you had an agreement with wasn't a mother. Motherhood makes you another person. I know that now. I didn't know it then'" (370).

Partially because of their genre and partially because of their choice of focus, the popular media do not show us what we are allowed to see in the novel—the deep depression Trudy descends into after giving up her child. For days she does nothing but stare at the walls, reliving the birth of her child. She won't eat; she runs a fever. The distraught Sinclair cannot pull her out of it. "It occurs to me that Sinclair is trying to cheer me up. . . . His flowers are lost now in the immensity of the darkness within me, specks of confetti ground into the asphalt" (375).

Just as the technology of *Brave New World* comes uncannily close to that of the real world, the birth situations in *The Handmaid's Tale* and *The Mommy Club* could have come from the popular media. Diedre Hall describes herself grabbing the baby boy from the surrogate before the cord was cut. Like the handmaids, Hall's surrogate "came from God with our name on her." The "hovering" girlfriend-type relationship Hall claims to have with the surrogate is just the type of relationship that Hillary has tried to cultivate with Trudy. Trudy, who has been contemplating keeping her baby since the ultrasound, is reminiscent of Anna Johnson, the surrogate who lied about her past pregnancies and who changed her mind before the baby was born. Her motivation is also one which has been cited by surrogacy brokers. Guilty over a past abortion (Sinclair's child), she made a deal with the baby that she would find a way to have him later on. In fact, for the sake of a happy ending, the realism of the *Mommy Club* must be cast aside. Sister Theonella has given the baby to Trudy's former roommate to care for, knowing she will come for her; Trudy reunites with Sinclair after a ten year hiatus; Sinclair happens to have $83,000.00 in savings, and Trudy comes out of her depression and realizes that she must retrieve her baby. She walks away from the Goettlers without even the hint of a custody suit. (Victor is both the biological father and a rich and powerful lawyer so one would expect some trouble from this quarter.) The novel ends with Sinclair singing the lines of a song:

> Wooo, life could be a dream, sh-boom,
> If only all my precious plans would come true,
> If you would let me spend my whole life loving you,
> Life would be a dream, sweetheart. (389)

All three of these novels succeed in calling attention to attitudes underlying technology that the popular media have eliminated or avoided. In the name of progress, *Brave New World*'s engineered society has edited out all of the pursuits that make life an adventure: art, science, philosophy, religion. When these are lost, a primal ingredient of humanity is lost: passion. The Savage cannot comprehend life without Shakespeare, God, or a reason for chastity. "'What you need,' the Savage went on, 'is something *with* tears for a change. Nothing costs enough here'" (162). He claims the right to be unhappy with all of its attendant problems and strongly-felt emotions. The Controller's world is one of comfort and convenience, of stability and certainty, but it is totally devoid of passion and humanity. The Savage's only choice is to commit suicide.

The Handmaid's Tale works out the logical conclusion of valuing women for their reproductive capabilities. When Offred describes herself and her colleagues, she says "[w]e are two-legged wombs, that's all: sacred vessels, ambulatory chalices" (176). The handmaids are told they are valuable, honored, but they can just as easily be declared "Unwomen" and sent to clean up nuclear waste. It is what is in the chalice that is sacred—male sperm. The handmaids' uteruses are the only valued part of them: "They didn't care what they did to your feet or your hands, even if it was permanent. Remember, said Aunt Lydia. For our purposes your feet and your hands are not essential" (118). At worst, the position the handmaids hold in the houses is extremely uncomfortable; the wives are hostile to them. At best they are well-treated servants, expected to be pure, pious, domestic, and submissive. Offred imagines how a simpering sell-out like Ofwarren might be treated: "Such a, so well behaved, not surly like some of them, do their job and that's that. More like a daughter to you, as you might say. One of the family" (147).

Finally, the handmaids are simply functional wombs who, if they fail, will be declared Unwomen, and if they succeed will be moved on to a new "posting," their identities obliterated once more and replaced with a new patronymic. "I am a blank, here, between parentheses. Between other people" (295).

Trudy is also a sort of servant. "I listen to the sounds of a house where I am not quite a guest, not quite a servant" (123). Recognizing this, and that she will be monitored constantly as soon as Hillary knows she is pregnant, Trudy manages to avoid telling her until she is in her fourth month. "'Fourth month?" she [Hillary] echoes, looking at me, horrified by my deficiencies in folic acid, iron, and calcium, to say nothing of simple record-keeping'" (97). When Trudy meets Victor for the first time, she tries a little humor to break the ice, and jokingly says "So you're the sperm donor" (74). These words echo Mary Beth Whitehead-Gould's characterization of William Stern. The comment clearly inverts and subverts the relationship the Goettler's prefer and Trudy must quickly cover for her gaffe: "'The firm loner," I corrected myself. "You're the *firm loner*, up here all alone'" (74).

Hillary's attitude toward motherhood is also worrisome. "'Parenthood,' she likes to tell me, 'is mostly a matter of organization. It's a time management problem'" (24). To "practice" staying home, she has their dinners catered "in." She attends a "Power of Myth class" at the Jung Center so that she can "liberate [herself] from the child within" (27). When she sizes up Trudy as a prospective surrogate, Trudy imagines her deciding that with Victor's genes and an "enriched atmosphere" they can overcome Trudy's genetic handicaps (50). For Hillary, having a child is simply a matter of "good housekeeping," a cross between managing a schedule, cultivating a plant, and practicing psychobabble. Perhaps it has been gleaned from the pages of a women's magazine?

Huxley's 1932 warning is about the potential of science to sever the natural relationship between sexuality and childbearing; it is about the dangers of allowing a small group of people to uncover all of the mysteries—mental and physical—that make us human. His tale is placed far into the future because, from his perspective in the 1930s, it would be a while yet before we developed the technology to carry out these practices. The effect of placing this novel so far into the future is to make its events seem less likely to happen and therefore less threatening. We can label it a dystopia and enjoy the fantastic quality of the events. By the end of the next decade, however, Huxley realized that science was moving at a faster clip than he had anticipated. "Then I projected it six hundred years into the future. Today it seems quite possible that the horror may be upon us in a single century" (xiv).

By placing her tale in the very near future, Atwood makes her world and its threats more possible, more frightening. Her Huxley-style warning is closer to home, harder to ignore. But Sarah Bird's tale *is* today. Trudy's story could have come from a newspaper account (though it would have been the story of the custody fight). This world defines not just the possible but the real, and it is now. The brave new world is upon us and we must recognize and deal with the dangers that are already occurring "inadvertently, from the best intentions" (Calder 12).

NOTES

1. This quotation was taken from *The Oxford Dictionary of Quotations*. 3rd edition. Oxford: Oxford University Press, 1979. 383.

CHAPTER SEVEN

Gynecology in the Future

The brave new world of reproductive technology has been ushered into the last half of the twentieth century due in part to the very understandable desire of a nineteenth-century doctor to bring practical experience to his readers. To include practical discussions in his textbook, Bard had to break taboos against male intervention into the intensely personal and private relationship that women had with the mysteries of birth. Though the gynecological case history was not born at this time, a new role for it was beginning. Within the context of the gynecology textbook, the case history played an important role in promoting that branch of medical science; once it found its way into the popular media, it began to serve as a representative anecdote that deflects rather than reflects reality. In the women's magazine, the case history paints a rosy fantasy world with "happy endings." In the commentary journal, the case history becomes the impetus for a critical debate of the problems posed by technology. In the news media, the case history is given a cursory examination that allows the introduction of both the miracle metaphor and the critical discussion into the text of our culture. Even the literary case histories we explored are not true representative anecdotes, for they highlight only the problems with this technology, leaving out those happy endings we saw so many of in the women's magazines.

The case history has helped science to unravel the mysteries of birth by promoting reproductive technology and creating clients for the infertility doctor/gods of the last half of the twentieth century. As we move into the twenty-first century, with the assistance of the case history, the powerful natural role that women have played in regenerating the species is subject to any manner of change.

Though it remains to be seen whether motherhood is a relationship that can truly be contracted out, it has already been fragmented by modern reproductive technologies. It is possible now to be a genetic mother, a gestational mother, and/or a social mother. In some cases, a child could have all three. This fragmentation is often supported in the accounts we have read of surrogacy arrangements and it is a fragmentation that will change the definitions of motherhood and parenthood. For the right price, a woman can now become a mother without interrupting her career—or ruining her figure. This would seem to signal complete liberation for women. However, where there is a social mother waiting in the wings, there is a gestational mother doing the work. The fact that other women must be used for this procedure reifies class distinctions between women; some are still valued for their ability to gestate, a definition feminists have worked very hard—perhaps too hard—to overcome. The case history often edits out the work that the gestational mother performs, leaving us looking at only the smiling faces of the social mothers who profit from their labor.

Writing about the full scope of reproductive technologies now available, Gena Corea gives us the real life case history of a sow when she describes her life in what she calls a "reproductive brothel." "It consists of pregnancy, birth, watching her babies being taken from her to be fattened for market, and then, endlessly, a repetition of the cycle: pregnancy, birth, loss of babies, insemination" (41). Comparing this description to human situations sounds harsh, but when Corea reports on the attitudes held by those in control of the industry we can see the potential parallel to contract mothers. She quotes the export development manager for a meat company: "'The breeding sow should be thought of, and treated as, a valuable piece of machinery whose function is to pump out baby pigs like a sausage machine'" (Taylor qtd. in Corea 41).

We may believe that women would never be treated this way, but our examination of case histories shows otherwise. Offred's position as a part of a great rotating reproductive brothel is no different really than the sow's. She is told repeatedly of her value as a "natural resource." If Atwood's novel still appears to be too fictitious to be taken seriously, then we must consider the surrogate mothers like Mary Beth Whitehead-Gould who have tried to make their voices heard about how it feels to have their babies taken from them. Or we can pay attention to people like William Handel by comparing his statement about the contract mothers who work for him—"'I scare the hell out of them'" (qtd. in Kasindorf 16)—with one that Gena Corea quotes from social commentator Vance Packard: "in South Texas 'pleasant conscientious Mexican-American girls' might leap at a fee of $5000 for bearing a child and girls [sic] south of the border might leap at half that fee" (43). The stage has already been set for abuse and the players are already in place, their lines memorized. The small drama that is the case history rehearses these scenes for the public in many venues. In some, like the women's magazine, it does so in a way that makes the drama of reproductive technology seem perfectly acceptable.

As medical technology "advances" even further we will one day have artificial wombs. At this point, the uterus will no longer be of value, but eggs will. Ovary harvesting will probably be the next step and we can be sure that a practice like this will be presented as a new "service" for women. Case histories like the one profiling Jeniffer the egg donor will praise the convenience that such a service will offer. This new case history will promote removing ovaries so women can stop worrying about becoming pregnant at an inopportune time. By donating most of their eggs, which they will never use anyway, women will be able to reserve space in an artificial womb for the time when they decide to have their own children. Will any woman then be allowed to gestate her own children or will case histories present this option as an obscene act, as in *Brave New World*?

The gynecological case history is also evolving; it has already entered the medium of television. We are now seeing these "miraculous" stories of birth on the movie of the week, soap operas, and on hourly news magazines. Television coverage is just as likely to exclude important considerations as that of the print media. We know that the woman who served as Diedre Hall's surrogate used the movie made from Mary Beth Whitehead-Gould's experience to convince her children that she should gestate a child for Hall. Certainly Gould would object to her story being used in this way.

A recent "60 Minutes" segment profiled a woman its writers labeled as a "go between." She procures egg donors for people and one of the scenes shows her sitting at the kitchen table with two women, one a prospective buyer, the other a prospective donor. They are looking at pictures of the prospective donor's children to get an idea of how the egg will perform. This comfortable little scene enacts the "catalogue of clones" scenario suggested by Elmer-DeWitt in the *Time* magazine article discussed in chapter five.

A more telling scene in the "60 Minutes" telecast is an interview with the egg procurer in which she confesses to having had her doubts about the ethics of her profession. She explains that she lost sleep at nights worrying about the egg donors she had located. The doctors were giving them very high doses of the fertility drugs to ensure a bumper crop of eggs. Her brow wrinkles as she explains her concern about working with unscrupulous doctors. By worrying over the doctor's ethics, the woman has avoided examining the practice of egg donation itself, and her role in this practice. Apparently she has found ethical doctors with whom to work and is again sleeping at night.

We will continue to be bombarded by the reprospeak that Robyn Rowland claims softens us up to technologies we might otherwise object to. The only defense against this indoctrination is to understand those messages and their underlying ideologies. The future of reproductive technology is potentially frightening, and we owe it to our children to pay attention to the rhetoric of its sales tactics.

I would like to conclude this discussion by presenting my reworded version of Burke's "Definition of Man." Mine has been adapted to represent the position woman inhabits in the gynecological case history:

> Woman is
> The symbolic surrogate (incubator and inculcator),
> Negated in her symbolic absence,
> Detached from her natural function by the tools of technology (made pious and pure by technology),
> Dominated by her sense of domesticity (or motivated by a sense of altruism),
> Motherhood in fragmentation.

Works Cited

Adler, Jerry, Mary Hager, and Karen Springen. "Clone Hype." *Newsweek* 8 November, 1993: 60-62.

Allegretti, Joseph. "Reproductive Technology Invades the Divorce Court." *America* 27 October 1990: 304-305.

Ames, Katrine. "And Donor Makes Three." *Newsweek* 30 September, 1991: 60-61.

Andrews, Robert. Ed. *The Columbia Dictionary of Quotations.* N.Y.: Columbia University Press, 1993.

Annan, Mrs. A. M. F. "Baby-Visiting." *Godey's Magazine and Lady's Book* December 1844: 266-273.

Arthur, T. B. "I Will!" *Godey's Magazine and Lady's Book* May 1844: 213-215.

Atwood, Margaret. *The Handmaid's Tale.* 1985. N.Y.: Fawcett Crest, 1987.

Baker, Nancy C. "The Secret of Our Very Special Baby." *Ladies' Home Journal* August 1980: 46-54.

Bard, Samuel, M.D. *A Compendium of the Theory and Practice of Midwifery.* 1st ed. N.Y., 1807.

Bard, Samuel, M.D. *A Compendium of the Theory and Practice of Midwifery.* 5th ed. N.Y., 1819.

Bazell, Robert. "In Vitro Veritas." *The New Republic* 15 February 1988: 11-13.

Begley, Sharon. "Little Lamb, Who Made Thee?" *Newsweek* 10 March 1997: 52-59.

Bird, Sarah. *The Mommy Club.* N.Y.: Laurel-Dell, 1992.

"Birth-Marketing." *Commonweal* 4 December 1987: 692.

"Bishop responds to embryo, abortion cases." *The Christian Century* 28 August 1996: 808-809.

Blakely, Mary Kay. "Surrogate Mothers: For Whom Are They Working?" *Ms.* March 1983: 18-20.

Blyth, Myrna. "Editor's Journal." *Ladies' Home Journal* January 1982: 2.

Bransford, Helen. "Surrogacy: A Mother's Story." *Vogue* July 1995:134-137+.

Brown, Clifton. "Of Family, and an Improbable Road to Parenthood." *New York Times* 25 December 1997, sec. C: 1+.

Brownlee, Shannon. "The Baby Chase." *U. S. News and World Report* 5 December 1994: 84-93.

Bruni, Frank. "The Gods of Fertility." *New York Times* 8 July 1998, sec. B: 1+.

Burke, Kenneth. *A Grammar of Motives.* 1945. Berkeley: University of California Press, 1969.

———. *A Rhetoric of Motives.* 1950. Berkeley: University of California Press, 1969.

———. *Language as Symbolic Action: Essays on Life, Literature, and Method.* Berkeley: University of California Press, 1966.

Calder, Jenni. *Huxley and Orwell:* Brave New World *and* Nineteen Eighty-Four. Studies in English Literature 63. Southampton, Great Britain: The Camelot Press, Ltd., 1976.

Callahan, Sidney. "Lovemaking & Babymaking: Ethics and the New Reproductive Technology." *Commonweal* 24 April 1987: 233-239.

Challender, Debbie. "Fertility Fraud: Why One Mother May Never Know Her Babies." *Redbook* December 1995: 84-87+.

Chesler, Phyllis. "What is a Mother?" *Ms.* May 1988: 36-39.

Chomsky, Noam. "The Bounds of Thinkable Thought." *The Progressive* October 1985: 28-31.

Cimons, Marlene. "Ratio of Multiple Births in U. S. Has Risen 214 Percent Since 1980." *Houston Chronicle* 29 January 1997: 12A.

Clark, Matt. "Infertility: New Cures, New Hope." *Newsweek* 6 December, 1982: 102-110.

Clifford, Cheryl, (with Mary Garner Ganske). "'God gave us four miracles.'" *McCall's* March 1997: 52-57.

Cohen, Cynthia B. "'Give me children or I shall die!': New reproductive technologies and harm to children." *Hastings Center Report* March 1996: 19-27.

Collins, Linny. "Debby prayed for a miracle—and got four!" *Woman's World* 22 March, 1994: 54-55.

Corea, Gena. *Man-Made Women: How New Reproductive Technologies Affect Women.* Bloomington: Indiana U.P., 1987.

Cutter, Irving S. and Henry R. Viets. *A Short History of Midwifery*. Philadelphia: W.B. Saunders Company, 1964.

Davidson, Arnold E. "Future Tense: Making History in *The Handmaid's Tale*." *Margaret Atwood: Vision and Forms*. Ed. Kathryne Van Spanckeren and Jan Garden Castro. Ad Feminam: Women and Literature. Carbondale: Southern Ill. U.P., 1988.

Davenport, Christine and Donna Freedman. "Oh baby, baby, baby, baby!" *McCalls* April 1995: 82-83.

deHolguin Cayzer, Bea. "Kim Casali's Miracle Baby." *Good Housekeeping* November 1977: 90+.

De Lee, Joseph B. A.M., M.D. *The Principles and Practices of Obstetrics*. 6th ed. Philadelphia: W. B. Saunders Company, 1936.

Del Zio, Doris and Suzanne Wilding. "I Was Cheated of My Test-Tube Baby." *Good Housekeeping* March 1979: 135+.

Delepine, Joy. "*Good Housekeeping* Gave Us Our Son." *Good Housekeeping* August 1982: 40+.

Delloff, Linda Marie. "The Noblest Baby of Them All." *The Christian Century* 14 July 1982: 749-750.

D'Emilio, Frances. "Mama mia! Italian woman, 62, becomes oldest to give birth." *Houston Chronicle* 19 July 1994: 12A.

Dilley, Becki and Lori Erickson. "Cuter by the Half Dozen." *McCall's* March 1998: 56-62.

"Divorced Couple is Awarded Joint Custody of 7 Embryos." *New York Times* 14 September 1990, sec. A: 20.

Eberlein, Tamara. "Too Many Babies? The Dangerous Rise of Multiple Births." *Redbook* August 1996: 88-91+.

Edmiston, Susan. "Whose child is this?" *Ladies' Home Journal* November 1991: 234-237+.

Edmondson Gupta, Nelly. "Brave New Baby." *Ladies' Home Journal* October 1989: 141+.

Edwards, Margot and Mary Waldorf. *Reclaiming Birth: History and Heroines of American Childbirth Reform*. N.Y.: The Crossing Press, 1984.

Efron, Sonni. "A 3-Way Fight for Custody." *Los Angeles Times* 3 March 1991: A3+.

———. "Surrogate Is Legal Mother, Judge Decides." 19 April 1991: A3+.

Elmer-Dewitt, Philip. "Cloning: Where Do We Draw the Line?" *Time* 8 Nov. 1993: 65-70.

———. "The Cruelest Kind of Fraud." *Time* 2 December, 1991: 27.

———. "Making Babies." *Time* 30 September, 1991: 56-63.

Evans, Sara M. *Born for Liberty: A History of Women in America.* N.Y.: The Free Press, 1989.

Fein, Elaine. "Love (times) 5." *Family Circle* 10 August 1993: 96-98.

"Fertility Clinics: What Are The Odds?" *Consumer Reports* February 1996: 51-55.

"53-year-old gives birth to grandson." *Houston Chronicle* 30 December 1992: 5A.

"The First Test-Tube Baby." *Time* 31 July, 1978: 58-69.

Fitzgerald, Kevin T. "Little lamb, who made thee?" *America* 29 March 1997:3.

Flynn, Eileen. "Fashioning the wanted child." *Commonweal* 14 March 1986: 148-150.

Footlick, Jerrold K. "Test-Tube Bereavement." 31 July, 1978: 70.

Fraser, Laura. "A Leap of Faith." *Good Housekeeping* March 1998: 110-111+.

Gaffney, James. "Hagar & Her Sisters: Precedent For Conduct." *Commonweal* 24 April 1987: 240-242.

Gallagher, Maggie. "Womb To Let." *National Review* 24 April 1987: 27-30.

Garvey, John. "Contracting Anguish: Sara, Melissa, Or Baby M.?" *Commonweal* 24 April 1987: 232.

———. "The seven McCaugheys." *Commonweal* 19 December 1997:7.

Garvey, Mark. Ed. *Writer's Market.* Cincinatti, Ohio: Writer's Digest Books-F.& W. Publications, 1993.

Gewertz, Catherine. "Surrogate's Custody Fight Opens." *Los Angeles Times* 10 October 1990: A3+.

———. "Surrogate Gives Birth to Boy, Custody Fight." *Los Angeles Times* 20 September 1990: A3+.

———. "Surrogate Mother Sues to Keep Couple's Child." *Los Angeles Times* 14 August 1990: A1+.

———. "Surrogate Mother's Visitation Rights Reduced by Judge." *Los Angeles Times* 28 September 1990: A34.

Gianelli, Diane M. "Senate kills anti-cloning bill, citing research concerns." *American Medical News* 2 March 1998:8.

Gladwell, Malcolm and Rochelle Sharpe. "Baby M Winner." *The New Republic* 16 February: 15-18.

Goodman, Ellen. "Toddler Needs a Parent, Not Legal Limbo." *Houston Chronicle* 21 September 1997: 6C.

Gordon, Linda. "Why Nineteenth-Century Feminists Did Not Support 'Birth Control' and Twentiety-Century Feminists Do: Feminism, Reproduction, and the Family." *Rethinking the Family: Some Feminist Questions*. Ed. Barrie Thorne and Marilyn Yalom. N.Y.: Longman, 1982. 40-53.

———. "Reproductive Rights for Today." *The Nation* 12 September 1987: 230-232.

———. "Voluntary Motherhood: The Beginnings of Feminist Birth Control Ideas in the United States." *Women and Health in America.* Ed. Judith Walzer Leavitt. Madison, Wisconsin: The University of Wisconsin Press, 1984. 104-116.

Gordon, Mary. "'Baby M'": New Questions About Biology and Destiny." *Ms.* June 1987: 25-28.

Gorman, Christine. "How Old Is Too Old?" *Time* 30 September, 1991: 62.

Greenblatt, Stephen Jay. *Three Modern Satirists: Waugh, Orwell, and Huxley.* New Haven: Yale U.P., 1965.

Gustaitis, Rasa. "infertility hype." *Glamour* March 1989: 76-84.

Gwynne, Peter. "All About That Baby.: *Newsweek* 7 August, 1978: 66-72.

Hall, Deidre, (with Lamanna, Dean). "What We Did For Love." *Ladies' Home Journal* December 1995:74-80.

Hellegers, Andre and Richard McCormick. "Unanswered Questions On Test Tube Life." *America* 19 August 1978: 74-78.

Hoffman, Jan. "Egg Donations Meet a Need And Raise Ethical Questions." *New York Times* 8 January 1996, sec. 1:1+.

Huxley, Aldous. *Brave New World.* 1939. Bantam-Grosset & Dunlap, Inc. N.Y.: 1968.

———. Introduction. *Brave New World.* 1946. By Huxley. Bantam-Grosset & Dunlap, Inc. N.Y.: 1968.

"Infantrepreneurs." *Commonweal* 19 April 1985: 228-229.

"In Iowa, the Birth of a Nation." *Newsweek* 29 December 1997: 66.

Jackson, Rosemary. *Fantasy: The Literature of Subversion.* New Accents. N.Y.: Methuen, 1981.

Johnson, Maureen. "British Scientists Destroy Thousands of Embryos." *Houston Chronicle* 2 August 1996: 20A.

Kalb, Claudia. "How Old Is Too Old?" *Newsweek* 5 May 1997: 64.

Kane, Elizabeth. "Sisters in Pain." *Redbook* April 1988: 114-115.

Kantrowitz, Barbara. "Who Keeps 'Baby M'?" *Newsweek* 19 January, 1987: 44-49.

Kasindorf, Martin. "And Baby Makes Four." *Los Angeles Times Magazine* 20 January 1991: 10-14+.

Katz, Bill and Linda Sternberg Katz. *Magazines for Libraries.* 6th ed. N.Y.: R.R. Bowker-Reed, 1989.

Kennedy, David M. *Birth Control in America: The Career of Margaret Sanger.* Yale Publications in American Studies, 18. New Haven: Yale U.P., 1970.

Keerdoja, Eileen. "Test-Tube Triumphs." *Newsweek* 6 December, 1982: 110.

Kerber, Linda K. *Women of the Republic: Intellect and Ideology in Revolutionary America.* The Institute of Early American History and Culture. Virginia: The University of North Carolina Press, Chapel Hill, 1980.

Kershner, Kelly. "In Vitro Fertilization: Is Conceiving a Child Worth the Costs?" *USA Today* May 1996: 30-32.

Kluger, Jeffrey. "Will We Follow The Sheep?" *Time* 10 March 1997: 66-72.

Kobrin, Frances E. "The American Midwife Controversy: A Crisis of Professionalism." *Sickness and Health in America: Readings in the History of Medicine and Public Health.* 2nd ed. Ed. Judith Walzer Leavitt and Ronald L. Numbers. Madison, Wisconsin: University of Wisconsin Press, 1985. 197-205.

Kolata, Gina. "Clinics Selling Embryos Made for 'Adoption.'" *New York Times* 23 November 1997: A1.

Kolata, Gina. "Cloning human embryos raises range of ethical, practical issues." *Houston Chronicle* 24 October 1993: 4A.

———. "Giving Older Women A Shot at Motherhood." *New York Times* 28 October 1990, sec. 4: 4.

———. "On Cloning Humans, 'Never' Turns Swiftly Into 'Why Not.'" *New York Times* 2 December 1997: A1+.

Krauthammer, Charles. "The Ethics of Human Manufacture." *The New Republic* 4 May 1987: 17-21.

Lacayo, Richard. "In the Best Interests of a Child." *Time* 13 April, 1987: 71.

———. "Whose Child Is This?" *Time* 19 January, 1987: 56-58.

Lait, Matt. "Family Experts Criticize Ruling in Surrogacy Case." *Los Angeles Times* 28 September 1991: A31.

———. "Judge Orders Co-Custody in Surrogate Case." *Los Angeles Times* 27 September 1991: A3+.

Lawson, Carol. "Couple's Own Embryos Used in Birth Surrogacy." *New York Times* 12 August 1990, sec. 1: 1+.

Leavitt, Judith Walzer. "Birthing And Anesthesia: The Debate over Twilight Sleep." *Women and Health in America.* Ed. Judith Walzer Leavitt. Madison, Wisconsin: The University of Wisconsin Press, 1984. 175-184.

Lee, Felicia R. "Infertile Couples Forge Ties Within Society of Their Own." *New York Times* 9 January 1996: sec 1:4+.

Lemonick, Michael D. "It's a Miracle." *Time* 1 December 1997: 34-39.

Lenhart, Jennifer. "Calls flood in on 'womb for rent.'" *Houston Chronicle* 16 November 1993: 17A.

Libman Block, Jean. "God Willed It." *Good Housekeeping* January 1979: 62+.

Liebmann-Smith, Joan. "Medical Miracle. . .Or Baby Selling?" *Redbook* November 1992: 120+.

———. "Two Friends with One Dream." *Redbook* March 1989: 122-123.

Lowry, Katharine. "The Designer Babies Are Growing Up." *Los Angeles Times Magazine* 1 November 1987: 7-12+.

Margolis, Maxine L. *Mothers and Such: Views of American Women And Why They Changed.* Berkeley: University of California Press, 1984.

Markoutsas, Elaine. "Women Who Have Babies for Other Women." *Good Housekeeping* April 1981: 96+.

Martin, Malachi. "Test-Tube Morality." *National Review* 13 October 1978: 1285.

May, Lee. "Estranged Wife Awarded Custody of Frozen Embryos." *Los Angeles Times* 22 September 1989: A1+.

McCormick, John and Barbara Kantrowitz. "The Magnificent Seven." *Newsweek* 1 December 1997: 58-62.

McDowell, Janet Dickey. "Ethical Implications of In Vitro Fertilization." *The Christian Century* 19 October 1983: 936-938.

McDowell, Jeanne. "Miracle Babies." *For Women First* 17 May, 1993: 30-34.

McKinney, Betsy Marvin. "The Pleasure of Childbirth." *Ladies' Home Journal* April 1949: 116+.

Meigs, Charles D., M.D. *Obstetrics: The Science and the Art.* 3rd ed. Philadelphia: Blanchard and Lea, 1856.

Melendy, Mary, M.D., Ph.D. *Perfect Womanhood for Maidens-Wives-Mothers.* N. p.: K.T. Boland, 1903.

Messer, Ellen and Kathryn E. May, Psy.D. *Back Rooms: An Oral History of the Illegal Abortion Era.* N.Y.: Touchstone-Simon & Schuster, 1988.

Meyers, John A. "A Letter from the Publisher." *Time* 21 July, 1978: 2.

Mills, Karen. "I Had My Sister's Baby." *Ladies' Home Journal* October 1985: 20+.

Mohr, James C. *Abortion in America: The Origins and Evolution of National Policy, 1800-1900.* N.Y.: Oxford University Press, 1978.

Morrill, C., M.D. *The Physiology of Woman, and Her Diseases* N.Y.: William T. Hamilton, 1856.

Morantz, Regina Markell. "Making Women Modern: Middle-Class Women and Health Reform in Nineteenth-Century America." *Women and Health in America.* Ed. Judith Walzer Leavitt. Madison, Wisconsin: The University of Wisconsin Press, 1984. 346-358.

———. "The 'Connecting Link': The Case for the Woman Doctor in 19th-Century America." *Sickness and Health in America: Readings in the History of Medicine and Public Health.* 2nd ed. Ed. Judith Walzer Leavitt and Ronald L. Numbers. Madison, Wisconsin: University of Wisconsin Press, 1985. 161-172.

Mydans, Seth. "Science and the Courts Take a New Look at Motherhood." *New York Times* 4 November 1990, sec. 4: 6.

Nash, J. Madeline. "All in the Family." *Time* 19 August, 1991: 58.

Neuhaus, Richard John. "The Return of Eugenics." *Commentary* April 1988: 15-26.

Neumann, Peter J. "Should health insurance cover IVF? Issues and options." *Journal of Health Politics, Policy & Law* October 1997: 1215-1239.

Neumann, Peter. J., Soheyla Gharib, and Milton C. Weinstein. "The cost of a successful delivery with in vitro fertilization." *New England Journal of Medicine* 28 July 1994: 239-243.

Nevins, Barbara. "The $2,000 Egg." *Redbook* November 1992: 118+.

Novak, Michael. "Buying & Selling Babies: Limitations On the Marketplace." *Commonweal* 17 July 1987: 406-407.

Nowakowski, Patty. "How Could I Let Them Separate My Twins?" *Redbook* July 1990: 38-41.

The Oxford Dictionary of Quotations. 3rd edition. Oxford: Oxford University, 1979.

Pancoast, S. M.D., and C.C. Vanderbeck, M.D., PH. D., *The Ladies' New Medical Guide*. Philadelphia: John E. Potter & Co., 1890.

Pollitt, Katha. "The Strange Case of Baby M." *The Nation* 23 May 1987: 667+.

———. "When Is A Mother Not A Mother?" *The Nation 31 December 1990: 825+.*

Post, Stephen G. The Judeo-Christian case against human cloning." *The Nation* 21 June 1997: 19-22.

Press, Aric. "Troubling Test-Tube Legacy." *Newsweek* 2 July, 1984: 54.

Pressley, Sue Anne. "It's a boy, girl, boy, girl, boy, girl, oh boy!" *Houston Chronicle* 20 November 1997: 1A.

Radovsky, Vicki Jo. "Special Report: Overcoming Infertility." *For Women First* 17 May, 1993: 37-38.

Raymond, Janice G. "Women as Wombs." *Ms.* May/June 1991: 28-33.

Redbook Research. N.Y.: Hearst Corporation, 1994.

Remsberg, Bonnie. "She is a Miracle." *Ladies' Home Journal* January 1982: 75-77+.

Richards, Louise. "Giving the gift of life." *Ladies' Home Journal* February 1989: 22+.

Rigney, Barbara Hill. *Margaret Atwood.* Women Writers. New Jersey: Barnes & Noble: 1987.

Roberts, John. "US doctors accused of misusing embryos." *British Medical Journal (International)* 2 September 1995: 585.

Rock, Andrea. "The Triplets Club. *Ladies' Home Journal* March 1996: 144-147.

Rosenblatt, Roger. "Baby M.—Emotions for Sale." *Time* 6 April, 1987: 88.

Rothman, Barbara Katz. "High-Tech Baby-Making: The Next Front Page Scandal?" *Glamour* June 1992: 210+.

Rowland, Robyn. *Living Laboratories: Women and Reproductive Technologies.* Bloomington: Indiana U.P., 1992.

Safford, Henry B., M.D. "Tell Me Doctor." Part 7. *Ladies' Home Journal* September 1950: 31+.

———. "Tell Me Doctor." Part 8. *Ladies' Home Journal* September 1950: 31+.

———. "Tell Me Doctor." Part 9. *Ladies' Home Journal* October 1950: 31+.

———. "Tell Me Doctor." Part 10. *Ladies' Home Journal* November 1950: 31+.

———. "Tell Me Doctor." Part 11. *Ladies' Home Journal* December 1950: 31+.

Saur, Mrs. Prudence. *Maternity: A Book for Every Wife and Mother.* Chicago: Monarch, 1896.

Scholten, Catherine M. "'On The Importance Of the Obstetric Art': Changing Customs of Childbirth in America, 1760 to 1825." *Women and Health in America.* Ed. Judith Walzer Leavitt. Madison, Wisconsin: The University of Wisconsin Press, 1984. 142-154.

Schweitzer, Arlette and Kathryn Casey. "My children, My grandchildren." *Ladies' Home Journal* February 1992: 125-127+.

Seaman, Barbara, and Gideon Seaman, M.D. *Women and the Crisis in Sex Hormones.* N.Y.: Rawson Associates Publishers, Inc., 1977.

Seligmann, Jean. "Five Years of Hard Labor." *Newsweek* 6 December, 1082: 108.

Sellers, James. "Test-Tube Conception: Troubling Issues." *The Christian Century* 16 August 1978: 757-758.

Simpson, Kevin. "Four little angels answered their prayers." *Woman's World* 12 July 1994: 12-13.

60 Minutes. CBS. KHOU, Houston. 7 August 1994.

60 Minutes. CBS. KHOU, Houston. 2 October 1994.

Sowers, Leslie. "Baylor Team Improves In Vitro Odds." *Houston Chronicle* 25 August 1996: 4D.

"The Sperm Bank Scandal." *Newsweek* 26 July, 1982: 24.

Squire, Susan. "Whatever Happened to Baby M?" *Redbook* January 1994: 60+.

Stockham, Alice B., M.D. *Tokology: A Book for Every Woman*. Chicago: Sanitary Publishing Co., 1884.

"Surrogate-gate." *Commonweal* 30 January 1987: 35-36.

"Surrogate loses her appeal." *Modesto Bee* 9 October 1991: B5.

Speert, Harold, M.D. *Obstetrics and Gynecology in America: A History*. Baltimore: Waverly Press, Inc., 1980.

Tagliabue, John. "In Italy, a Child Is Born, And So Is a Lively Debate." *New York Times* 13 January 1995, sec. A: 8.

"The Tangled Web of Surrogacy Issues." *Los Angeles Times* 28 September 1991: B5.

Templeton, Allan, Joan K. Morris, and Willliam Parslow. "Factors that affect outcome of in-vitro fertilisation treatment." *Lancet* 23 November 1996: 1402-1406.

"Test-Tube Babies." *Commonweal* 1 September 1978: 547-548.

Travaglini, Kris. "Our Miracle Daughter." *Ladies' Home Journal* May 1992: 24-28.

Ulrich's International Periodical Directory. 32nd ed. vol. 2 Bowker, 1993.

"Vatican says mom defied will of God." *Houston Chronicle* 20 July 1994: 16A.

Venn, Alison, Lyndsey Watson, Judith Lumley, Graham Giles et al. "Breast and ovarian cancer incidence after infertility and in vitro fertilisation." *Lancet* 4 October 1995: 995-1000.

Walker, Susan. "Why I became a single mother." *Ladies' Home Journal* March 1985: 22-24.

Warren, Susan. "Sign gives pregnant pause." *Houston Chronicle* 13 November 1993: 1A+.

———. "Surrogate no stranger to state, federal agencies." *Houston Chronicle* 19 November 1993: 1A+.

———. "Womb lessor called sweet and friendly." *Houston Chronicle* 22 November 1993: 11A+.

Warren, Susan and Bob Sablatura. "'Womb-for-Rent' woman in trouble with law." *Houston Chronicle* 18 November 1993: 1A+.

Welter, Barbara. "The Cult of True Womanhood, 1820-1860." *Women and Womanhood in America*. Ed. Ronald W. Hogeland. Lexington, Massachusetts: D.C. Heath and Company, 1973. 103-114.

Wertz, Dorothy C. "Man-Midwifery and the Rise of Technology: The Problem and Proposals for Resolution." *Birth Control and Controlling Birth: Women Centered Perspectives.* Ed. Helen B. Holmes, et al. New Jersey: Humana, 1980. 147-167.

"What makes a parent?" *Glamour* November 1991: 48.

White, Robert J. "Human Embryo Research." *America* 14 September 1996: 4-5.

Williams, Linda S. "No Relief Until the End: The Physical and Emotional Costs of In Vitro Fertilization." *The Future of Human Reproduction.* Ed. Christine Overall. Toronto: The Women's Press, 1989. 120-139.

Williams, Maureen Smith. A "Quint-essential" Christmas. *McCall's* December 1988:107-109.

Williams, Patricia J. "I a child, and thou a lamb." *The Nation* 2 February 1998: 8.

Wilt, Judith. *Abortion, Choice, and Contemporary Fiction: The Armageddon of the Maternal Instinct.* Chicago: University of Chicago Press, 1990.

Woloch, Nancy. *Women and the American Experience.* N.Y.: Alfred A. Knopf, 1984.

Wood, James Playsted. *Magazines in the United States.* 2nd ed. N.Y.: The Ronald Press Company, 1956.

Yates, Laurie and Jean Libman Block. "Don't take my babies from me!" *Good Housekeeping* March 1988: 115+.

Zophy, Angela Marie Howard. "For the Improvement of My Sex: Sarah Josepha Hale's Editorship of *Godey's Lady's Book, 1837-1877.*" Diss. The Ohio State University, 1978.

Index